Fertility, Cycles and Nutrition

Can what you eat affect your menstrual cycles and
your fertility?

Marilyn M. Shannon

Important Notice

This book describes various relationships between diet, nutrition, body balance and fertility. It has been written as a general educational guide and reference for both concerned individuals and health care professionals.

While this book accurately represents the findings of much research, it cannot be considered a "prescription" for any person with any particular situation. Neither the author nor the publisher can assume medical or legal responsibility for the use of this book or its information by individuals or health care professionals. You will find it carefully documented so that interested parties can readily pursue further research.

Persons with symptoms of illness should seek diagnosis and care from competent physicians and/or other licensed health care professionals.

Fertility, Cycles and Nutrition

Can what you eat affect your menstrual cycles and your fertility?

Marilyn M. Shannon

The Couple to Couple League International, Inc.
Cincinnati, Ohio 45211

Cataloging data.

Dewey: 612.32
L. C.: 90-82244

Shannon, Marilyn M.

Fertility, Cycles and Nutrition: Can what you eat affect your menstrual cycles and your fertility?

1. Nutrition   2. Health, reproductive
3. Menstrual cycles   4. Natural family planning
5. Infertility   6. Pregnancy

Acknowledgements

Thanks go first to John F. Kippley, a founder of the Couple to Couple League for Natural Family Planning. Having the privilege of teaching natural family planning through this organization for the past eight years has sparked my interest in the relationship between nutrition and reproductive health, and it was he who suggested that I undertake this project.

Special thanks go to my husband Ron, who not only invented the "80-20" rule (Part I, Rule 12) but who has also provided the moral support necessary for a homeschooling, expectant mother of four to find the time involved in researching and writing this book.

I gratefully acknowledge the assistance of Dr. Douglas Wartzok, Chairman of the Department of Biological Sciences of Indiana University-Purdue University at Fort Wayne, in providing the resources necessary to produce the original manuscript. Many thanks go to Mrs. Sandra Fisher of the same department, who typed the first draft, and to Mrs. Betty Schwartz of the Couple to Couple League, who typed the many revisions.

I am indebted to Edward M. Keefe, M.D., of Greenwich, Connecticut, and to Arlene F. Smith, D.O., of Lansing, Michigan, for their critical reviews of the manuscript. All errors, however, are my own responsibility.

Thanks are due Mrs. Jane Dawkins of Fort Wayne, Indiana, who prepared Tables 4 and 7. Finally, I wish to express my gratitude to those men and women who shared with me their experiences with nutrition and reproductive health. Their anecdotes are contained within these pages.

Grateful acknowledgement is also given for the following materials:

Quoted material on pages 85, 86 and 88 is reprinted from *Prevention's Medical Care Yearbook 1989*, ©1989 by Rodale Press, Inc. Permission granted by Rodale Press Inc., Emmaus, PA 18098.

The quoted materials on pages 92 and 93 are excerpts from *Vitamin B₆: The Doctor's Report*, ©1973 by John M. Ellis and James Presley. Reprinted by permission of Harper and Row, Publishers, Inc.

The quoted material on page 101 is reprinted from *Let's Have Healthy Children,* by Adelle Davis, revised by Marshall Mandell, M.D., ©1981 by The New American Library.

The quoted material on pages 114-115 is reprinted from *How To Be Your Own Nutritionist,* by Stuart M. Berger, M.D., ©1987 by the author. Reprinted by permission of William Morrow & Co.

The quoted material on pages 119-120 is reprinted from *The Yeast Connection,* by William G. Crook, M.D. ©1983, 1984, 1985, 1986 by William G. Crook, M.D. Reprinted by permission of Random House, Inc.

The quoted material on page 137 is reprinted from *The Right Dose*, ©1987 by Rodale Press. Permission granted by Rodale Press, Inc., Emmaus, PA 18098.

Table of Contents

Foreword

I cannot recall how or when it first dawned on me that there was a connection between nutrition and fertility, but once that dawning occurred, I saw increasing evidence of it as I counseled couples—and especially women—about natural family planning. When a woman has a reasonably normal fertility-menstrual cycle, the practice of natural family planning (NFP) is simple, and the amount of abstinence is quite limited. However, if a woman has menstrual periods that drag out to seven, eight or even ten days, one sort of difficulty is encountered. Again, if ovulation is delayed and the mucus sign of fertility continues for quite some days, additional abstinence is required by those using NFP to postpone or avoid pregnancy. On the other hand, I have seen couples seeking pregnancy become even more frustrated when ovulation occurs only three or four times per year or when they fail to achieve pregnancy within a few *apparently* normal cycles.

What we have discovered is that many of these difficulties can be overcome or alleviated by improved nutrition or body condition. Let me share two anecdotes that illustrate my convictions.

1. One of our teachers of natural family planning called me about her newly-irregular cycles. She had always had quite normal cycles, but just recently ovulation was being delayed considerably. She had started to diet and had stopped consuming any salt. That meant she had eliminated the most likely source of iodine which is necessary for the proper functioning of the thyroid gland. I suggested she take one kelp tablet each day as an iodine supplement. She did so and immediately returned to clockwork cycles.

2. A young engaged woman was having very long cycles with an extended time of apparent fertility. She gave no

appearance of being anorexic, but she had been a competitive swimmer during college and still swam perhaps five times a week. By this time I knew something about the importance of the fat to muscle ratio (body balance), and I shared a bit of that. She reduced her swimming somewhat, stayed the same weight, and developed perfectly normal length cycles. The most plausible explanation is that she increased her fat to muscle ratio sufficiently to bring about normal fertility cycles.

Marilyn Shannon has had similar and even more dramatic cases in her counseling. Our collective experience leads us to this conclusion:

IN MANY CASES, CYCLE IRREGULARITIES CAN BE EITHER ELIMINATED OR ALLEVIATED SIMPLY BY BETTER NUTRITION OR BODY BALANCE.

In making that statement, we are using "cycle irregularities" to cover a multitude of situations which are spelled out in Part II of this book. It also applies to certain aspects of male fertility and even to birth defects and repeated miscarriages.

Marilyn Shannon has rendered a great service to women in general and to NFP couples in particular by writing this book. The information was out there—buried in the scientific journals. She put it all together in one readable book. I am personally very grateful to her for the great service she has rendered in making the research available to be applied by ordinary people.

The purpose of this book is to help readers understand how to assist the natural fertility processes to function normally through good nutrition. What is unique about this book is that this is the only resource I know of that addresses so many "female problems," a couple of "male problems," and infertility in terms of nutrition. It then offers suggestions on how to achieve or maintain normality through proper nutrition and body balance.

The bottom line of this book is threefold: through improved nutrition and/or body balance—

1) Many women will be able to have more normal fertility-menstrual cycles;

2) Many marginally fertile couples seeking pregnancy will find increased fertility;

3) Many couples will find it much easier to practice natural family planning.

I might add that this book is going to make the work of many NFP counselors—including myself—much easier.

— John F. Kippley, President
The Couple to Couple League International, Inc.
Cincinnati, Ohio

Introduction

Couples who are already practicing a healthy lifestyle, including emphasis on holistic nutrition, are often drawn to the practice of natural family planning (NFP). Conversely, those who choose NFP primarily for other reasons often seem to broaden their interests to include more natural approaches to other areas of life and health. For example, interest in alternative childbirth options is high among NFP users, and the rate of breastfeeding is simply phenomenal. Success in the practice of natural birth regulation, without recourse to chemicals, devices or surgery, undoubtedly encourages such couples to take further responsibility and to work in harmony with their physical selves in other areas such as nutrition.

There are some striking parallels between natural family planning for birth control and holistic nutrition for health or healing. Both may be termed "appropriate technology" in that they rely on the intelligent use of ordinary things (food, vitamins, information) that may be obtained without undue effort or expense. As such, they are all too often overlooked in an environment in which the high technology of synthetic pharmaceutical agents or surgery are frequently the unthinking first choices for birth control or health care. Both NFP and nutrition require for their success a certain amount of personal commitment, bodily self-awareness and discipline of the appetites, either sexual or for food. Yet both offer large rewards for these small sacrifices—and a major one is improved physical health over the long term.

Within the medical community, natural family planning for child spacing and nutrition for prevention and healing of illness share a similar position. Both are insufficiently taught in medical schools; consequently, the typical medical doctor is generally unaware of their value and is frequently unhelpful when asked for advice in either area. In the last several years, however, laymen's groups (such as the Couple to Couple League for Natural Family Planning, La Leche League International, and the publishers of *PMS Access*) have become recognized as leaders in disseminating information about their respective specialties. Interestingly, though, it is the exceptional medical doctors who *are* interested in and knowledgeable about these two areas who have provided the scientific validity and clinical experience which make such lay efforts possible.

Despite the close kinship between NFP and nutrition, a real gap has existed in relating the two for practical applications. While natural family planning may be practiced successfully despite a wide range of reproductive disorders, experience shows that couples are happier with it when the times of abstinence are not prolonged by various cycle irregularities and when the use of the infertile times is not disrupted by premenstrual syndrome (PMS), prolonged menses, vaginal infections or the like. For couples using NFP to overcome infertility, excellent nutrition is as essential as the charting of fertility signs and the timing of intercourse. Information from the medical literature concerning nutritional aids for these and other problems certainly does exist, but it has been fragmented, difficult to locate, and to a great extent simply buried in the research journals in medical libraries. With the single exception of the nutritional strategies for PMS, such information has been greatly underestimated in its value.

This small book is intended to close the "information gap" between natural family planning and nutrition for reproductive health. The first part, "Good Nutrition for Good Health," reflects my belief that good nutrition is the best health protector, whether we are referring to reproductive health, cardiovascular health or any other aspect of health. You may notice, in fact, that these dietary recommendations are similar to those that are now suggested to prevent cardiovascular disease, some types of cancer, and a host of digestive disorders. The "high fiber-low fat" diet based on a wide variety of whole foods seems simply to be the diet on which human beings thrive with the least problems for the longest time.

The second part tackles specific reproductive problems, starting with PMS. Since PMS shares a common cause with several other disorders, it is recommended reading even for those who are free from it.

Part III contains some ideas for continuing to help yourself. "Finding a Nutritional Counselor" addresses the issue of professional guidance when it comes to nutrition. Just as NFP requires learning and counseling, so does nutrition, especially when used for healing. The "Further Reading" and "Resources" pages again emphasize the role of individual responsibility; there is no substitute for your own informed awareness of the often controversial new ideas that are currently transforming the world of nutrition.

Part I

Good Nutrition
for
Good Health

The highest priority for maintaining good health is nutritious food. Almost every thoughtful person agrees on this point, yet many of us have not yet made the changes necessary to eat properly. Perhaps this is because our food preparation methods and our taste for various foods are so deeply ingrained through culture and habit. They certainly resist dramatic change! Envisioning better nutrition as meals composed of such unfamiliar items as tofu or adzuki probably discourages many homemakers who really would like to improve their family's diet.

The encouraging news is that drastic alterations in the foods we eat are not necessary, and the much-maligned American diet can actually be used as the foundation for excellent nutrition. Good nutrition is far more a matter of careful selection and emphasis than wholesale change from, say, meat and potatoes to soy-oat patties. By practicing the following rules of thumb, we can greatly increase the value of our family's meals while we continue to "cook American."

1

Twelve Rules for Improved Nutrition

Rule 1: Eat more complex carbohydrates, less saturated fats, and adequate, not excessive, protein.

Proportion makes an immense difference to our nutritional status. Americans are notorious for their emphasis on animal fats and proteins and their neglect of the "complex carbohydrates." The latter term refers to every variety of edible grain, seed, nut, root or other plant part; these foods should comprise well over fifty percent of our daily calories. Overall fat intake should not exceed thirty percent of our daily calories and, ideally, should be closer to twenty percent. The saturated fat sources—meat, dairy products, shortening, and processed peanut butter—should be limited, but small amounts of the beneficial unsaturated oils such as safflower, soy, canola, peanut and olive oil should be taken in daily. Unless protein needs are high due to pregnancy, lactation or physical exertion, animal protein should be used in modest portions.

A special word about fats. Most of us are aware that consumption of excess saturated fat and cholesterol is unhealthy. Many people, though, are unaware that other types of fat are beneficial to health and even contain factors which are essential to life itself. The polyunsaturated oils contain linoleic acid, an essential factor. Safflower oil, sunflower oil and corn oil are polyunsaturated, but converting the latter to shortening (hydrogenation) results in a saturated product in which the beneficial linoleic acid is destroyed. The same result occurs when soy oil is hydrogenated to make margarine. The monounsaturated fats, found in olive oil, canola oil and natural peanut butter, also contribute importantly to the normal balance of fat metabolism in the body. As with shortening, the hydrogenation of processed peanut butter saturates it, destroying the very monounsaturated oils which make it so valuable a food.

Rule 2: Substitute more nutritious ingredients for less nutritious ingredients.

Nutritionally inferior ingredients are those that contain avoidable saturated fats or white flour, added salt, sugar, artificial colors or preservatives. These are usually found in prepackaged or processed foods which provide mostly empty calories and insufficient vitamins, minerals and fiber. Their additives may also act as toxins in the human body. Table 1, "Foods to Limit," lists such foods.

Table 1
Foods to Limit

Sugar	Processed cheese
White flour	Excessive butter or
Fruit juices	margarine
Soft drinks	Excessive salt;
Prepackaged foods	uniodized salt
Fatty meats	Aluminum-containing
Bacon, sausage, wieners,	baking powder
lunch meats, ham	Coffee
Shortening	Chocolate
Processed peanut butter	Caffeine-containing tea
Artificial food additives,	Excessive dairy products
including aspartame	
(Nutrasweet)	

More nutritious foods are simply leaner, fresher, and closer to their natural state. Whole natural foods are rich in the "micronutrients"—vitamins and minerals—and the highly beneficial fiber has not been refined away. Since they do not contain additives, they minimize the problem of harmful chemicals. Their natural starches and sugars are slowly released to the blood, maintaining steady blood glucose levels. Table 2, "Foods to Emphasize," lists such foods, and Table 3, "Food Substitutions," gives examples of more nutritious foods which can easily be used in place of nutritionally inferior foods in your familiar recipes and dishes.

Table 2
Foods to Emphasize

Fresh fruits
Fresh vegetables
Whole grain breads
Whole grain pasta
Brown rice, millet
Whole grain flours
 (Barley, rice,
 buckwheat, soy)
Dried beans
Natural peanut butter
Nuts and edible seeds

Unsaturated oils, such as
 safflower, soy, canola,
 peanut or olive
Lean meats
Poultry
Liver, heart (in moderation)
Milk (in moderation)
Yogurt
Eggs (in moderation)
Herbal teas

Rule 3: Eat more raw foods, and cook other foods gently.

Heating food kills bacteria and parasites, makes the food easier to digest and makes certain nutrients more available. It also destroys vitamins. For example, several B vitamins and vitamins C and E are all harmed by cooking. As much as possible, fruits should be eaten raw, not cooked or juiced. Vegetables which need cooking can be briefly steamed or heated in a little boiling water. Fish and meat should be prepared at low temperatures and cooked just long enough for good taste and safety.

Table 3
Food Substitutions

Use	Instead of
100% whole grain bread	White bread or "wheat" bread
Whole wheat and small amounts of whole grain flours (rice, barley, buckwheat, or soy)	White flour
Brown rice or millet	White rice or instant rice
"Old-fashioned" rolled oats	Quick-cooking oats
Granola	Packaged breakfast foods
Bran muffins	Sweet rolls
Whole grain noodles	White flour pasta
Sweet potatoes, acorn squash, butternut squash, turnips	White potatoes
Dark green vegetables	Light green vegetables
Romaine lettuce, spinach, leaf lettuce, bibb lettuce, endive or escarole	Iceberg lettuce
Fresh vegetables	Frozen vegetables
Frozen vegetables	Canned vegetables
Deep yellow or orange vegetables	Light yellow or white vegetables
Whole fruits	Fruit juices
Homemade soups	Canned soups
Poultry, heart, liver or ocean fish	Red skeletal meats
Low-fat milk	Whole milk
Natural cheeses	Processed cheeses
Natural peanut butter	Processed peanut butter
Unrefined safflower, soy or canola oil	Shortening or corn oil
Low-calorie salad dressing with added safflower oil	Commercial salad dressing
Fruit-based desserts	Chocolate, sugar and cream desserts

Rule 4: Eat a greater variety of foods.

The best, freshest, most toxin-free natural food cannot

build health alone. Other than mother's milk for the infant, no complete food exists. The dozen or so basic foods that Americans eat—beef, milk, potatoes, white bread, and so forth—do not supply all of the dietary factors that produce optimal health. For example, the late eighties' discoveries of the healthful effects of the omega-3 unsaturated oils in fish and the possible cholesterol-reducing effect of soluble fiber illustrate that we have simply not discovered all there is to know about the factors that promote the best health. The greater the variety of nutritious foods we eat, the greater chance we have of acquiring all the beneficial dietary factors we need, including those as yet undiscovered. Table 4, "Minimum Daily Food Goals," is a checklist designed to encourage you to eat a wide variety of nutritious foods every day.

Rule 5: Sharply limit sugar and caffeine.

Table sugar, brown sugar and honey are all calorie-rich, micronutrient poor, and rapidly absorbed. When we snack on a candy bar or soft drink, especially on an empty stomach, the blood sugar is suddenly jolted upward. The pancreas reflexly reacts to this stress by secreting the hormone insulin. Insulin quickly lowers blood sugar levels by allowing glucose entry into the body cells (including the fat cells, where any excess is stored as saturated fat). When this blood sugar jolt is repeated again and again, the pancreas apparently overresponds. It becomes overly efficient, and the physiological insult of high blood glucose brought on by the rapid absorption of sugar results in insulin overproduction and low blood glucose levels in a short time. This is "reactive hypoglycemia." Its symptoms include fatigue, irritability, headaches, and the inevitable craving for more sugar.

Sugar also depletes the body of hard-to-get B vitamins, chromium, zinc, manganese and magnesium, all of which are necessary to metabolize it.[1] It lacks the important fiber found in unrefined carbohydrate foods. While naturally sweet fruits provide micronutrients and fiber, very sweet fruits such as ripe peaches, grapes and oranges may also trigger reactive

— continues on page 12

Table 4
Mimimum Daily Food Goals

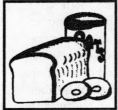

WHOLE GRAINS

3 servings daily (1 serving = 2 slices bread or 1/2 cup cooked cereal)

- Whole grain bread
- Oatmeal
- Whole grain breakfast cereal
- Whole grain pasta
- Whole grain pancakes
- Rice
- Millet
- Tortillas
- Bagels

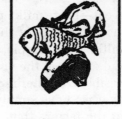

COMPLETE PROTEIN

1 serving daily (1 serving meat = 3-4 oz.)

- Poultry
- Fish (preferably twice weekly)
- Beef, including liver and heart
- Pork
- Lamb
- Grain + Legume (peas, beans, peanut butter, nuts, lentils)
- Dairy + Grain
- Dairy + Legume

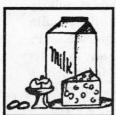

DAIRY/EGGS

3 servings daily (1 serving = 6 oz. milk, 2 oz. cheese, 1 egg)

- Milk
- Yogurt
- Cheese
- Ice cream
- Kefir
- Eggs

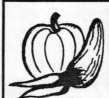

YELLOW FRUITS AND VEGETABLES

5 servings *WEEKLY* (1 serving = 1/2 cup cooked or 1 cup raw)

- Carrots
- Squash
- Sweet Potatoes
- Pumpkin
- Cantaloupe
- Apricots
- Peaches

Table 4, cont'd.

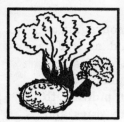

LEAFY GREEN VEGETABLES

2 servings daily
(1 serving =
1/2 cup cooked
or 1 cup raw)

- Lettuce (leaf, Romaine, bibb, iceberg)
- Spinach
- Escarole
- Endive
- Beet greens
- Alfalfa sprouts
- Cole crops (cabbage, broccoli, Brussels sprouts, cauliflower, kohlrabi)
- Asparagus
- Chard
- Kale

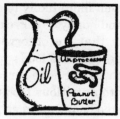

UNSATURATED OILS

1 serving daily
(1 serving =
1 - 2 tablespoons)

Polyunsaturated
- Safflower oil
- Sunflower oil
- Soy oil
- Corn oil

Monounsaturated
- Peanut oil
- Unprocessed peanut butter
- Olive oil
- Avocado oil

Both
- Sesame oil
- Canola oil

(Weekly intake should be approximately 50% polyunsaturated, 50% monounsaturated.)

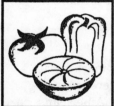

VITAMIN C SOURCE

1 serving daily
(1 serving = 1 medium fruit or 1/2 cup berries)

- Citrus fruits (oranges, grapefruits, tangerines)
- Tomatoes
- Melons
- Berries
- Peppers
- Potatoes

NOTES

- Each type of food should be counted only once per day.
- If you are pregnant or nursing, see Table 7.
- This table may be photocopied, covered with adhesive-backed clear plastic and taped to your refrigerator. Check off the boxes daily with an erasable marker.

hypoglycemia, especially on an empty stomach. Sweet fruit juices are even more likely to do so.

Sugar and honey do serve a useful role in encouraging us to eat foods that we otherwise probably would not. For example, the valuable foods yogurt and cooked oatmeal are rather grim without honey or jam. The goal should be to link sweeteners to nutritious foods—to bran in bran muffins, to beans in baked beans, to fresh greens in salad dressings, and so forth. My belief is that sugar is less harmful on a full stomach, so occasional treats should be desserts, not snacks. Honey is somewhat sweeter than table sugar and contains a few micronutrients, but the rule for all sweeteners should be the less, the better.

Caffeine directly affects the nervous system, causing anxiety, irritability and sleep disruption. It depletes the body of B vitamins and raises blood glucose by overstimulating the adrenal glands. The latter effect triggers the insulin response, ultimately causing hypoglycemia and the craving for more caffeine. Coffee is a well known source of caffeine, but cola, chocolate and nonherbal teas also contain caffeine or related compounds which have similar effects. Some over-the-counter medicines such as Midol and Anacin and a few cold remedies contain caffeine. Since this chemical also affects blood vessel constriction, it is best to eliminate caffeine consumption gradually over a period of two weeks or more to avoid withdrawal headaches.

Rule 6: Chew your food thoroughly.

This often-repeated, often-ignored advice has more merit than one might guess. In truth, it makes little difference with the typical overcooked, low-fiber diet that many Americans consume. But we are wasting the nutrients in raw or lightly cooked vegetables, grains and fruits if we wolf them down. Chewing thoroughly breaks the fiber away from the cells, releasing the vitamins and minerals. Look at it this way: these foods are too valuable to gulp!

Rule 7: Store natural foods carefully to minimize nutri-

ent loss and spoilage.

Processed foods have a longer shelf life than many natural foods because spoilage-prone parts have been refined away and artificial preservatives have been added. The refrigerator, freezer and covered plastic containers will more than compensate for this "problem" with whole foods. In particular, whole-grain flour, wheat germ, unsaturated oils, butter, and natural peanut butter must be covered and refrigerated to prevent rancidity. Dried grains and beans can be left at room temperature in canisters with tight-fitting lids—they are nutritious foods that will readily support insect life! Potatoes should be stored in the dark to prevent their turning green.

Rule 8: Beware of eating out.

Breaking all the rules occasionally at a fast food restaurant can be enjoyable, but for the person who must eat lunch or another meal away from home regularly, eating-out options present a formidable obstacle to improved nutrition. Fast food or cafeteria fare typifies the worst of American food—highly salted French fries, white buns, and soft drinks; or white noodles, greasy meats and endlessly overcooked vegetables.

Eating well before leaving home is an excellent strategy. Or bring a meal in a brown bag, or pack a snack of raw fruits, vegetables, seeds or nuts. Avoid the fries and soft drinks, and choose the fresh greens—not the canned fruits!—at the salad bars that many restaurants now feature. If vending machines are a particular temptation, resolve to carry no change, and bring a brown bag instead. It is interesting to note that excellent restaurants prepare their meals from gently handled fresh ingredients. You can certainly eat nutritiously at such establishments, especially if you choose small portions of meat. The price will increase your appreciation of your own nutritious, delicious meals.

Rule 9: Obtain pure drinking water if possible.

The Environmental Protection Agency reported in 1975 that over 250 organic compounds had been identified in

American tap water.[2] The problem of agricultural runoffs, industrial wastes and leaks is still serious, but the ability to acquire clean drinking water conveniently and reasonably has improved immeasurably.

Distilled water or water treated by reverse osmosis is thought to be the purest. Either can be obtained in many communities through home delivery (about $1.00/gallon in 1990 prices) or pick-up ($0.55/gallon), and the availability of water purified by reverse osmosis and sold inexpensively through conveniently located vending machines is spreading widely ($0.35/gallon). Supermarket distilled water is also inexpensive ($0.60/gallon), though the leaching of the soft plastic into the water raises questions in my mind. Home distillers ($300) or reverse osmosis units ($600-900) are expensive but effective answers to unsatisfactory tap water. Before you dismiss the idea of paying for healthful drinking water, consider the price of soft drinks—$1.20 to $8.00 per gallon.

Rule 10: Prepare your meals thoughtfully.

Nutritious, tasty, simple to prepare—these describe the ideal meal. So far we have dealt with the first without addressing the other two. But if we emphasize the principle of improving the ingredients of familiar dishes, we will already have one important element of good taste—familiarity. What is familiar is likely to be enjoyed. Moreover, the freshness, naturalness, and gentle cooking of nutritious foods will automatically add gourmet taste. Good foods taste good!

Once you eliminate the sugar added so liberally to packaged foods, you'll also discover that natural foods are often quite sweet. Constant consumption of soft drinks, baked goods and desserts stimulates rather than satisfies the sweet tooth. Conversely, when these are sharply reduced, the sensitivity to sweet taste markedly improves. The sweetness of carrots, of whole wheat bread, even of grapefruit will surprise you.

14

Simplicity is a major consideration, with so many home-makers so busy. The rule of thumb of using a greater variety of foods is of real value here. Many of the convoluted, time-consuming recipes that clutter our cookbooks are only an attempt to create variety where it doesn't exist. For example, it's easy to scrub and microwave a white potato. So why peel it, boil it, mash it, French fry it or au gratin it? Or beef: there are actually cookbooks with names like *101 Ways to Serve Hamburger!* Instead of depending on so many inconvenient ways to disguise the same old foods, offer real variety and prepare it simply.

Breakfast. The newest research, affirming the benefits of the complex carbohydrates, should convince us that the traditional breakfast based on cereal is still ideal. (By cereal I mean the generic term for grains, not the overadvertised junk foods also claiming that name!) Rolled oats, cooked oat bran, granola, bran muffins and multi-grain pancakes are all excellent foods. Whole wheat cereals are also nutritious, but wheat is so commonly used for bread that it is an excellent idea to avoid it in breakfast grains. Eggs are good, but not every day—moderation is in order for these cholesterol-loaded natural foods. Whole fruits offer freshness and fiber which are absent in fruit juices; prefer the fruit to the juice. Help yourself to the yogurt or have some milk, but skip the bacon and sausage for good.

Lunch. Lunch is great for sandwiches of whole grain bread packed with tuna salad, natural cheese, peanut butter, leaf lettuce, tomatoes and so forth. Soups, tacos, corn bread, yogurt, fruit, leftovers or perhaps another breakfast food such as multi-grain pancakes can expand the menu. Or microwave a sweet potato or squash for lunch. Keep it simple, and your children, like mine, will prepare it for you!

Dinner. If you are like most Americans, you probably prepare the evening meal around a protein and three complex carbohydrates. These carbohydrate dishes give us something to work with! Just reduce the amount of protein, and broaden your protein menu with ocean fish, poultry, liver or heart. Use the "potato position" for brown rice, millet, sweet potatoes, corn, squash or whole grain pasta. Then cook up a hefty serving of dark green vegetables—whatever is in season or on sale. Make your salad last but serve it first, and make it big!

Casseroles and stews are nutritious and economical ways to limit animal proteins and increase complex carbohydrates. Your favorites can be improved by substituting better ingredients for poor ones (Table 3) and adding the vegetables at the last minute.

I do not serve dessert with dinner except on special occasions. This not only eliminates extra sugar, but it also simplifies dinner preparation considerably. What foods take more elaborate preparation than those gooey cookbook desserts?

Snacks. The importance of snacks to certain individuals should not be underestimated. Children, pregnant and nursing mothers, and anyone who tends toward hypoglycemia (often characterized by extreme fatigue improved by eating, or migraine headaches in the morning or late afternoon) may find snacks just about a necessity. Complex carbohydrates and protein foods make the best snacks, because their nutrients are slowly digested and released over a long period of time. Milk, yogurt, whole wheat bread, seeds, nuts and granola cereal make good snacks. Simple sugars, including very sweet fruits, are the worst snack foods, since they cause wide swings in the blood glucose. Mothers of toddlers who wake up frequently at night or who resist bedtime may find that a hearty snack before bed solves the problem. Bedtime snacks may also help prevent morning headaches in some individuals.

Rule 11: Enlist your family's cooperation.

Make no mistake about it—if your spouse or children rebel at your efforts to improve the family's nutrition, it's an uphill battle. I have no specific advice for the recalcitrant spouse, other than to appeal to his maturity, reason and taste buds, but as the mother of four children, I feel qualified to offer some suggestions to encourage children to good nutritional habits and attitudes.

First, keep junk food out of the house. Children can then be permitted to choose their own breakfasts, lunches or snacks. A corollary to this is to avoid the television. There are better reasons than nutrition for doing so, but pulling the plug will also prevent your children from being tantalized by the shameless advertising of worthless foods.

Next, let the children participate in every phase of food preparation, from gardening to actual cooking. Then brag about it at dinner: "Rosemary picked the asparagus. John cooked the fish." The child who helps prepare the food is already prejudiced in its favor. I frequently set the table or act as "gofer" while my wonderful helpers, perched on stools, make salads, scrub vegetables, or cook pancakes. I also take the children shopping and have them select the fresh vegetables, seafood, and other items.

Actively teaching the children about nutrition is an immense aid. Of course, your own example is your best teaching aid; picky parents have pickier children! I recommend the school book, *Health, Safety, and Manners 3*, by Delores Shimmin.* This is a lovely Christian book suited to children from first to sixth grade. Only two of its chapters cover nutrition, but you and your children will enjoy the other chapters also.

If you have not had children yet, you can plan beforehand to get future babies off to an excellent start in nutrition, and save many problems later on. Sheila Kippley's wonderful *Breastfeeding and Natural Child Spacing** covers early solid feeding as well as the best nutrition, breastfeeding. I believe my children's enthusiasm for salads, rice, millet, fish and liver is an outgrowth of their early feeding. I have never used baby food; in fact, I have never even mashed my babies' foods, and I've never spoonfed them anything. I've let them feed themselves cooked broccoli, asparagus, carrots and so forth—why spoonfeed a baby who stuffs everything into his mouth anyway? I've concluded that pureed baby foods spoil a child's taste for textured food like salads and vegetables for years. And the recognizable beans and peas that inevitably appear in the diaper are probably nature's way of preventing the young

* *See "Further Reading"*

child from obtaining too much nutrition from adult food at the expense of his mother's milk.

Finally, strive for harmony at the dinner table. Such harmony has a value even beyond its role in family bonding. It is a real factor in our nutrition. Tension at the table, the American policy of "eat and run" or other unpleasantness stimulate the sympathetic division of the nervous system— the "fight-or-flight" division. Among the effects of sympathetic activity are inhibition of the digestive secretions necessary to chemically digest the food, and diversion of the blood supply away from the digestive organs. Thus, both efficient digestion and absorption of the digested food molecules from the intestines into the blood are inhibited when the sympathetic division is active.

On the other hand, a gracious mealtime followed by a bit of relaxation quiets the sympathetic nerves and encourages the parasympathetic division of the nervous system, stimulating all aspects of the digestive and absorptive processes. Body and spirit are truly inseparable! On a practical level, forcing children to eat disliked foods or sending them away from the table to punish lapses of manners is terribly counterproductive. These inevitable dinner table problems can be resolved at another time. The parents who set the tone of the dinner by inviting the Lord's presence and then complimenting their children on their salad making, table setting or pleasant manners are helping to nourish both body and spirit.

Rule 12: Use the "80-20" rule.

This means that we should sincerely attempt to make our diet 80% ideal. Having done that, we should not belabor the imperfect 20%. It simply is not realistic to commit the time and effort to locating and preparing organically grown foods of prime freshness all the time. Completely avoiding all junk food also restricts us from some of the most meaningful celebrations in our culture—birthdays, weddings, Christmas. And our children are far more likely to accept our leadership in matters of nutrition if they understand that we are reasonable; that treats are not forbidden—but that they are treats.

18

2

Acquiring Nutritious Food

The practical matter of actually obtaining the right foods is often the difference between whether or not we implement our nutritional goals. When nutritious ingredients have completely replaced refined foods in your home, it's easy to use them in the same dishes you have always served. And when your home contains no junk food, you can snack healthfully on whatever you choose from the refrigerator. The hurdle that many homemakers face, however, is to learn to acquire the best foods conveniently and economically.

If you are presently eating the worst of the American diet—too much meat, sweet baked goods, soft drinks, fatty foods and coffee—you can improve your nutrition immensely while still shopping at the same supermarket. But there are other sources of healthful foods which may offer better nutrition and sometimes lower prices. The following are thumbnail sketches of the nutritional possibilities of the supermarket as well as alternative food sources.

The Supermarket

It's obvious that the explosion of interest in holistic nutrition has paid off well for the consumer at the grocery store. Many whole, natural foods are now stocked in entire sections of the larger stores. Brown rice, whole grain pasta, barley, granola, safflower oil and natural peanut butter are commonly available. The variety of meats, ocean fish, and produce offered at most supermarkets is large and growing.

Even if a grocery store does not contain expanded sections of natural foods, it can still remain the basic place to shop. Experienced nutrition-conscious homemakers "shop the four walls." That is, they favor the basics—produce, meat, fish and dairy items—along the walls, ignoring the processed foods in the center of the store. Grains and beans for casseroles are the least expensive source of carbohydrates, and together they form complete protein. Liver and heart are low priced, compensating for the higher price of ocean fish. It is both nutritionally and economically sound to increase the variety of your fresh produce purchases by selecting whatever is in season or on sale.

The Health Food Shop

Good health food stores are actually miniature groceries which specialize in food supplements as well as organic and natural foods. It is helpful to understand these two terms before you purchase foods labeled as such. "Organic" refers to foods that are grown on mulched or manure-enriched fields without the use of chemical fertilizers, herbicides or pesticides. With reference to animal products, it means that the animal was fed from such land, and that no hormones or antibiotics were used. "Natural" means unprocessed. Thus "natural" millet has not been refined after harvesting, but it has been grown using conventional farming methods and chemicals. Organic foods are the Cadillac, and their price reflects the difference. They will contain more vitamins and minerals and less toxins than other foods.

Health food stores are generally more expensive than grocery stores, but they carry several desirable items not found in supermarkets—unrefined safflower, soy, and canola oils, iodized sea salt, aluminum-free baking powder, organic whole grain flours and pasta. You will also find a wide variety

20

of convenient breakfast cereals based on nutritious grains. They stock many whole grains, and some carry fresh-baked breads made with organic ingredients. Many feature organic produce.

If the nearest health food store is inconveniently far away or too expensive for your budget, at least use it to purchase unrefined vegetable oils, aluminum-free baking powder, iodized sea salt and whole grains, flours and pasta. The grains will keep indefinitely in canisters, and the flours can be frozen if necessary. I prefer the privately-owned health food shops to the typical shopping mall chains, since the former usually emphasize whole foods to a greater degree than the latter. Both, however, are far better sources of food supplements than are pharmacies.

The Food Co-op

Food co-ops typically sell a wider variety of natural and organic foods than the health food shops, and they offer reduced prices to members as a result of direct bulk purchasing and no-frills storekeeping. These are excellent places to buy your grains, beans, flours, oil, honey, bran, and pasta. Co-ops are a boon to those who wish to eat nutritiously on a shoestring budget. Members who work a few hours per month get additional price reductions on their purchases. I've seen mothers tending the counter while their toddlers played nearby in a toy-filled corner. Food co-ops also serve as an unofficial clearinghouse for alternative health care in your community; co-op employees are often able to recommend nutritionally-aware health practitioners, local midwives, and self-help groups for allergic individuals, PMS sufferers, and others.

Farmers' Markets

Are you aware that many cities feature wonderful farm markets where you can buy fresh produce brought in by nearby truck farmers? These markets are the next best thing to your own garden. The huge farmers' market in Milwaukee where I used to shop was filled with incredible bargains. We lived there as budget-conscious newlyweds, and my temptation was always to buy more than the two of us could possibly consume. These popular markets usually are open for a limited number of hours and days during the growing season only. Shop carefully and you will certainly find a wide variety of produce, gratifying freshness, and even organically grown items.

Gardening

Your own garden is good for the soul as well as the body, and it can be a wonderful family project. Give yourself a couple of summers to get good at it, and please don't invest in a tiller, herbicides or even a spade until you read *The Ruth Stout No-Work Garden Book** or other books by the late Ruth Stout. This author explains in a highly readable way the art of mulch gardening—using spoiled hay, straw, fall leaves or grass clippings to prevent weeds, retain moisture and fertilize the soil. Using a modified version of this method, we till our large garden less than once a year with a rented tiller. We do use small amounts of conventional fertilizer and the low-toxicity pesticide rotenone. We scarcely pull a weed.

My suggestion for beginners is to plant whatever grows the best with the least care. Tops on my list is asparagus. This hardy vegetable will produce for you the fourth year after planting, and will feed you scrumptiously and effortlessly for years early each spring while you're just putting in the spinach seeds! High fencing for tall pole beans and edible pod peas (Sugar Snap, an incredible raw treat) will maximize your yields and minimize your bending. Nothing is easier to grow than sweet corn, and nothing compares with ripe corn picked as the water boils.

Beets, turnips, lettuce, onions, broccoli, Brussels sprouts, cabbage and tomatoes are other easy-to-grow plants with high nutrient returns. I have no use for dwarf plants, which yield dwarf harvests. If space is truly limited, you will be happier with semi-dwarf fruit trees than with the shallow-rooted full

* See "Further Reading"

22

dwarfs. The easiest fruit of all to grow is the Concord grape which needs no spraying and thrives for years.

Private Farmers

The popularity of such magazines as *The Mother Earth News, Country Journal,* and *Organic Gardening* is evidence that there are growing numbers of families who own small amounts of land and are attempting to raise chemical-free vegetables, fruits, meat or dairy products. If you have the land to do this yourselves, by all means give it a try. If you're a young couple still not settled in your own home, I encourage you strongly to consider a few acres zoned for agriculture. If homesteading is already your dream, I sincerely hope you will make it come true.

If such an undertaking is out of the question, I can assure you that there are homesteaders around who would enjoy the extra cash of raising an antibiotic- and hormone-free lamb or steer for you. No, you don't end up with a four-footed potential steak in your suburban garage! They take the animal to a custom butcher, and you literally pick up the pieces, all cut and wrapped according to your specifications. Rabbit, goat, and chicken can be obtained in this way also. The first two may be unfamiliar but are quite lean and mild-tasting. We personally have traded our home-grown lambs for many things, and our children sell our organic eggs. There are other small farmers like us out there; you can contact them through the local advertising tabloids that are so popular everywhere.

Helpers in the Kitchen

Once you have acquired nutritious whole food, whether from grocery or garden, you will be storing it, preparing it and serving it. Many of the tools that are already in your kitchen are well adapted to these tasks. Others that you may not now own are also worth considering.

The **refrigerator** is basic, of course, and the bigger the better. Many natural foods must be refrigerated (Rule 7), and you'll need space for all your fresh produce. A **deep freezer** is especially useful for those who garden or raise their own meat. **Microwave ovens** make it easy to bake sweet potatoes, squash and other vegetables, and when combined with rapid-action yeast and glass bread pans, they reduce total bread-rising time to one hour.

Yogurt makers will save many dollars in yogurt. I own two and make enough yogurt at one time to last. I scald the milk in the microwave and use disposable styrofoam cups instead of the glass cups for added convenience.

Nothing will help you increase your raw food consumption like the Cuisinart **food processor**. It turns out huge amounts of green salads and cole slaw in seconds. It slices fresh beets, tomatoes, and stew vegetables. It also chops cold chicken for salad, tuna for tuna patties and potatoes for potato pancakes. It can be used to make peanut butter, mayonnaise, and vegetable oil pastry. It grinds meat for those who butcher their own animals. It's expensive (the Cuisinart DLC-7 Super Pro is $200 or more) but will repay you for years in big, fresh salads with minimal effort or cleanup. I have also noticed that the smaller pieces that it produces seem to help my young children really enjoy their salads.

A set of good-sized **salad bowls** is essential; if your salad fits on one edge of your plate, it's not big enough! Extra **canisters** are important for your brown rice, millet, barley, beans and whole grain pasta. **Pots** with tight-fitting lids are necessary to steam vegetables, and a really big soup pot is useful if there are to be leftovers. A **no-stick frying pan** and lecithin in liquid or spray form help you to avoid extra cooking oil in pan-fried foods. A **pressure cooker** is a great aid to bean cookery.

The right **cookbook** could be the most important "ingredient" for preparing healthful meals. The ideal cookbook should use all natural ingredients, it should provide lots of options so that recipes can be adapted to your taste or pantry supplies, and every single recipe must be quick and easy!

*Whole Foods for the Whole Family,** by La Leche League International, was written by and for busy mothers who wish to eat holistically while "cooking American." It not only meets all of the above criteria, but it has sections on making your own whole wheat bread, peanut butter, sprouts, yogurt and other nutritious foods. It explains how to cook brown rice, millet, dried peas and beans. I recommend that you cover it with clear plastic and treat it with care—mine is already grimy from overuse!

Finally, may I suggest something not directly related to food preparation? A beautiful set of **inexpensive china**. Yes, even if you, like us, have young children. A beautifully set table with a lovely tablecloth and centerpiece adds such graciousness to your meal and encourages you to prepare your best meals for your family as well as your guests.

See "Further Reading"

3

Supplements
to Consider

I believe that judicious use of vitamin and mineral supplements is a health practice second only to wholesome food in the benefits it provides. The purpose of this chapter is to explain the value of careful supplementation and to suggest a plan of micronutrient supplements which is within the limits of safety, comprehensive enough to be beneficial, and flexible enough to be tailored to your individual needs.

Why supplement? First, to overcome micronutrient deficiencies within the diet. The argument that additional vitamins and minerals are unnecessary if a "balanced diet" is eaten withers under scrutiny. Based simply on the wide genetic variation of humans and the definition of average, almost all of us are likely to have higher than average needs for one or more of the forty-odd essential nutrients. We may not absorb particular micronutrients well from the digestive tract, a problem that increases with age—even while caloric needs are decreasing. Many therapeutic drugs destroy vitamins; for example, some antibiotics destroy folic acid, and aspirin lowers levels of vitamin C, vitamin K and iron. Entire groups of individuals are known to have higher nutrient requirements than their "balanced diet" provides—nursing and pregnant women, dieters, smokers, drinkers, the elderly, oral contraceptive users, those who exercise vigorously and those with acute or chronic illnesses.

Secondly, when we consider our foodstuffs, the "balanced diet" becomes more illusion than reality. Vitamins and minerals are lost when foods are harvested in an under- or overripe state, when foods are stored, preserved, heated, peeled, juiced or even exposed to air. When only a limited variety of foods is eaten, the chance for adequate intake of every micronutrient diminishes further. Even our raw fruits and vegetables are not as nutrient-rich as they might be, since most are grown on eroding soils replenished with only a few minerals, and cultivated year after year. The domestic crops themselves are hardly "natural"—many have been extensively bred for traits such as high yield, uniform size, or sweet taste, not micronutrient content.

But how many of us are actually eating a "balanced diet" *on a daily basis?* The fantastic growth of the fast food chains tells a dismal tale; my experience as a college instructor of adults of all ages has driven home to me this point: many, many individuals habitually eat appallingly deficient diets.

Certainly another reason to consider supplements is to overcome specific health problems. The scientific literature contains numerous new studies demonstrating the salutary effects of specific nutrients on a wide variety of human illnesses. Part II of this book cites such studies involving reproductive disorders; the *Nutrition Almanac** also contains many citations of current research involving nutritional aids for other ailments. These studies are published in respected, peer-reviewed journals by medical doctors and other credentialed investigators; double-blind studies are well represented along with promising open studies.

Finally, judicious supplementation can help us toward the goal of optimal health. Optimal health refers to more than the absence of disease. It refers to a state characterized by abundant energy, emotional stability, and the ability to participate vigorously in life's work and recreation. While optimum health is a subjective condition, improved energy level and sense of well-being are common reports among supple-

* *See "Further Reading"*

ment users and undoubtedly contribute to their widespread and continuing popularity.

Among a growing number of health professionals, the real question is not whether to supplement but how to do so effectively and safely. The ideal is to provide the body with optimal levels of its essential nutrients while carefully avoiding toxicity and recognizing that unbalanced supplements can produce unanticipated nutritional deficiencies. Table 5, "Supplements to Consider," is a general plan for supplementing the micronutrients effectively, comprehensively and safely.

In many cases the suggested amounts of the vitamins and minerals in this plan are substantially higher than the well-known "Recommended Daily Allowances" (RDAs). RDAs are formulated to cover the minimal nutrient needs of the majority of healthy individuals and to prevent the classic deficiency diseases such as scurvy, beri-beri, pellagra and rickets. They are not geared to overcoming illnesses nor intended to represent optimal intake. Published reports of vitamins and minerals used to overcome specific physical disorders such as reproductive dysfunction seldom involve RDA levels of the nutrient in question.

The amounts of supplements listed in Table 5 are in the general range suggested by clinically experienced, nutritionally oriented physicians such as Guy Abraham, the well-published PMS researcher, Stuart Berger, a practicing physician, nutritional researcher and author, and other medical doctors whose writings are cited in this book. Among those who support the philosophy of optimal rather than minimal nutrition and among those who are implementing the new nutritional research, the suggested plan is rather conservative and without extremes of any single nutrient.

Far more critical than comparing supplement dosage to the rock-bottom RDAs is relating them to their toxic levels. The issue of vitamin and mineral overdose has been addressed admirably by Patricia Hausman, author of the *The Calcium Bible* and former staff nutritionist for the Washington, D.C., Center for Science in the Public Interest. She conducted an exhaustive search of the scientific literature to uncover all published reports of adverse reactions to vitamins and minerals. The results of this unique study are published in a practical form for the layman entitled *The Right Dose.** This is a fine reference for those concerned about the possibility of micronutrient overdose—which should be anyone who takes supplements. The author summarizes the literature on adverse reactions for each nutrient, includes an ample bibliography, and offers reasonable opinions as to the safe long-term upper limit for the supplements. In Table 5, I have included a very brief summary of "ceiling figures" or other cautions from this author. The *Nutrition Almanac* also contains information on vitamin toxicity, and Dr. Stuart Berger, in *How To Be Your Own Nutritionist,** uses his clinical and research experience to comment on adverse reactions to supplements which may occur in certain individuals, especially those with serious health disorders.

The following guidelines are offered to enable you to reap the considerable benefits of nutritional supplementation and to minimize the possible risks.

1) Proper diet is a higher health priority than supplementation. Supplements cannot compensate for a low-fiber, sugar-laden, or fatty diet.

2) Seek realistic nutritional counseling when you supplement. Part III of this book addresses this issue.

3) If you suffer from any serious disorder such as diabetes, liver, kidney or cardiovascular malfunction, make every effort to find a medical doctor who is aware of the specific risks *as well as the specific benefits* that supplements may hold for you.

4) Strive for balance when you supplement. High doses of some nutrients can cause depletion of or increased requirements for others. The B vitamins deserve special attention in this regard. While "balanced" B complex supplements in the

* See "Further Reading"

suggested amounts are readily available, tablets of the B vitamin folic acid of 1,000 micrograms (mcg; equal to 1.0 mg) or more are obtainable by prescription only. (Folic acid may mask vitamin B_{12} deficiency in strict vegetarians and those with gastrointestinal abnormalities.) In the higher potency B vitamin supplements, such as the 50 or 100 mg/mcg amounts, folic acid is far too low for balance, and should be taken separately in 400 or 800 mcg tablets which are widely available without prescription (see Table 5).

Other nutrients which must be properly balanced include calcium and magnesium; to take the former without the latter is to invite magnesium deficiency. Copper and zinc must also be balanced with one another. Vitamin A increases the need for vitamin E, and vitamin E's activity is enhanced by selenium. Calcium cannot be absorbed without adequate vitamin D. Nor is this an exhaustive list. Because of the interaction of nutrients and the need for balance, I strongly recommend that any program of supplementation include all of the essential nutrients listed in Table 5. *Even if research indicates that only one micronutrient has reversed a physical problem that you are attempting to overcome, this principle of balanced supplementation still holds true.*

5) Always take vitamin and mineral pills on a full stomach, preferably in divided doses after each meal. Increase and decrease supplements gradually, not abruptly.

6) Read supplement labels carefully. Ask for complete labels on prescription vitamins, especially prenatal vitamins, which are surprisingly low in potency. Pharmaceutical house multi-vitamins are closely tied to RDAs and are far less potent than the health food store brands, so my suggestion is to obtain as complete a multi-vitamin/multi-mineral supplement as possible from the latter. Even so, you will probably have to "round out" these supplements with additional folic acid, magnesium, vitamins C and E, and perhaps others.

7) Timed-release vitamins help to overcome urinary losses of supplements, and "chelated" minerals are more absorbable than other preparations of minerals. Both are worth the small extra cost.

Table 5
Supplements to Consider
Vitamins

Recommended Amount per Day		Comments on Safety*
A	5,000 - 20,000 I.U.	25,000 I.U. is conservative maximum except during pregnancy; use 20,000 maximum if pregnant.
B_1	25 - 100 mg	Toxicity rare.
B_2	25 - 100 mg	No toxicity reported.
Niacin (B_3)	25 - 100 mg	Known toxicity begins at 750 mg; use niacinamide, not nicotinic acid.
B_6	25 - 100 mg	Reported toxicity begins at 500 mg; consider nutritional counseling over 200 mg.
Pantothenic Acid	25 - 100 mg	No toxicity reported.
Choline	25 - 100 mg	May cause depression at much higher levels.
Inositol	25 - 100 mg	No known toxicity.
para-Aminobenzoic Acid (PABA)	25 - 100 mg	No data from Hausman.
B_{12}	25 - 100 mg	No toxicity reported; rarely, may mask folic acid deficiency.
Biotin	25 - 100 mg	No toxicity reported.
Folic Acid	400 - 2,000 mcg (0.4 - 2.0 mg)	May increase need for zinc; rarely, masks B_{12} deficiency in vegetarians and those with pernicious anemia. Relatively safe, even at 5,000 - 10,000 mcg. Requires vitamin C.
C	1,000 - 2,000 mg	Chewing may increase tooth decay. May decrease copper levels. Relatively safe except in iron-overload disease.
D	400 - 600 I.U.	The most toxic vitamin. 1,200 is threshold of toxicity.
E	400 - 800 I.U.	Considered safe at 1,000 I.U., even by its opponents; Hausman recommends 400 I.U. as a "good, safe dose."

Minerals

Recommended Amount per Day		Comments on Safety
Calcium	500 - 800 mg	Conservative long-term maximum is 1,500 mg.
Magnesium	500 - 1,000 mg	No toxicity reported from supplements. Avoid dolomite as source.
Iron	0 - 30 mg	18 - 30 mg/day is safe maximum. Iron overload must be considered.
Iodine	150 mcg	No date from Hausman; toxic at high levels.
Copper	2 - 3 mg	Toxic at high levels.
Zinc	25 - 50 mg	Excess zinc decreases copper; Hausman recommends 25 mg maximum.**
Manganese	10 mg	Low toxicity.
Potassium	from diet	No toxicity reported for over-the-counter preparations.
Chromium	150 mcg	No known toxicity at this level.
Selenium	50 - 200 mcg	500 mcg is safe maximum for total intake — diet plus supplements.

* From Hausman, P., 1987, The Right Dose, New York: Ballantine Books. In all cases, these comments refer to long-term supplementation in individuals without serious health disorders. If liver, kidney, cardiovascular or other such disease is present, consultation with a nutritionally-aware physician is essential.

** Zinc is so valuable for overcoming infertility and other reproductive dysfunctions that I hesitate to limit the suggested supplement amount to 25 mg as Hausman suggests. I have opted instead to accept the opinion of Stuart Berger, M.D., who considers 75 mg optimal and 150 mg the maximum safe dose (Berger, S., M.D., 1987, How To Be Your Own Nutritionist, New York: Avon Books, 348).

4

Questions and Answers

• What is the best way to get more of the beneficial oils in my diet?

First, realize that heating an oil damages its valuable fatty acids, so frying foods in oil is emphatically not the way to increase your oil consumption. My favorite trick is to add unrefined safflower or soy oil to commercial low-calorie salad dressing—shake it up and pour it over your salad. Or make your own salad dressings. That way the oil isn't heated.

Nutrition experts now recommend that half our oil intake be polyunsaturated (corn, safflower, sunflower, soy) and half be monounsaturated (peanut, olive, avocado). Sesame and canola oils are naturally "half and half." Natural peanut butter is a convenient source of peanut oil, and when you get down to the "clayey" solid part at the bottom, moisten it with safflower or soy oil. Olive oil has a zippy taste that you may enjoy on your salad or in spaghetti sauce. Use it to prevent pasta from sticking after you cook it. Aim for a tablespoon or two total oil per day—don't overdo. Incidentally, oil can and should be substituted for shortening in virtually every recipe you use, except for truly irredeemable concoctions such as ladyfingers. I've never had shortening in my kitchen for any of my thirteen years of marriage, and I haven't missed it yet.

- ## Which is preferable, butter or margarine?

Less of either is better than more of either. Health food store margarines made with soy oil are probably the best. Or you can whip together soy oil with softened butter in a 1:2 ratio—refrigerate (or freeze for longer storage) to prevent separation. I know others feel strongly about this issue, but I don't. I do suggest you use a *salted* butter or margarine, because the salty taste is probably what you're after anyway, and you'll use less if it is present.

- ## What is millet? How do I use it?

Millet is an exceptionally nutritious, fiber-rich grain that is an excellent source of B vitamins and magnesium. It's a staple in many parts of the world. You may recognize it as bird seed—those round, little yellow seeds that many bird feeds feature. It cooks exactly like rice (one cup of grain to two cups of water or so, bring to a boil, cover, simmer for about half an hour) and can be used in any recipe that calls for rice. Its flavor is mildly reminiscent of lima beans, but like rice, you eat it with a sauce. It's good with Chinese dishes, as chicken and "rice," and in stuffed peppers. Cook extra and refrigerate the rest to use later in multi-grain pancakes, along with oatmeal, wheat bran, whole wheat and other flours.

- ## I'm overwhelmed when I think of giving up caffeine and sugar. I don't really know where to start.

Don't plan on giving them up; instead, plan on cutting down on them. A really good idea is to promise yourself that you will have them only after a full meal, or only after a nutritious, fiber-rich snack followed by a big glass of cold water. This will almost automatically reduce the amount of these that you eat or drink, and it will also limit the swings in blood sugar that create the craving for more. And do not underestimate the value of unsaturated oils and fiber in satisfying your appetite and thereby reducing cravings for unhealthful snacks.

I certainly consider eating a good diet a higher nutritional goal than taking supplements, but in this case I think starting supplements a week or two before you begin to break your sugar and caffeine habit will make it easier to change. This is so because certain micronutrients tend to regulate blood glucose levels. "Hypoglycemia" in Chapter 5 mentions specific nutrients which may help to reduce these cravings by improving blood glucose control.

• I don't think I can afford supplements. Any thoughts about their expense?

Good vitamins *are* more costly than "one-a-day"-type vitamins based on RDAs. I personally feel that "time is money"; that is, the extra productive time I have because of the added energy they give me is well worth the monetary investment. I took this question to a friend of mine, a divorced mother of three young children who works only part-time for their sake. She is on the tightest budget of anyone I know, but she always serves holistic food to her family. She replied:

I buy health food store vitamins before I buy anything else. It's my highest priority for off-budget items. I can't afford to be sick, or miss work, or miss school. My kids and I hardly ever get sick any more. I'd be sick four or so times a year with the flu before I took vitamins.

As the admen say, good nutrition doesn't cost, it pays. For many of us, though, insurance and paid sick leave mask the true financial cost of poor nutrition.

• What kind of vitamins should young children take?

My opinion is that nursing babies and toddlers are fine with the vitamins they get through their mother's milk, assuming she supplements, as even those who are usually prejudiced against supplements recommend. For older children, health food stores have chewable vitamins. Strictly avoid vitamins with food colorings in them. Ask your nutritional counselor for specific recommendations because children at different ages need proportionally more of some micronutrients and less of others. Their systems are more effective at absorbing nutrients than are adults', and if I had to choose between supplements for a child or providing supplements for an adult, I'd choose the adult every time, assuming both are eating a reasonably good diet and both are in reasonably good health.

• **I have four small children, and even though they're good kids, I feel constantly "stressed out" by the sheer amount of work around the house. Can nutrition make a difference? I don't see how I can slow down.**

The well-nourished person can perform a tremendous amount of work, day in and day out, without reaching "wit's end." Cutting out caffeine is the first step because it contributes to that anxious feeling. The mineral **magnesium** is probably the most noticeably nerve-calming nutrient, followed by the **B vitamins**. Calcium supplemented without magnesium is especially detrimental as it may cause nervousness and anxiety. The nutritional strategies for keeping blood sugar up really help to give you the energy to tackle the day's activities—see Rule 5 in Chapter 1 and the discussion of hypoglycemia in Chapter 5. **Vitamin E** may also boost your energy.

I know that many people would suggest that you hire household help for this common problem, but the price of one morning's help can buy you a month's supply of vitamins. I'd choose the latter without hesitation, though I do not intend to diminish the role of diet, exercise and adequate rest. The physical stress of multiple pregnancies, nursing, of being on your feet constantly and being "on-call" twenty-four hours a day—it's incomprehensible to me that anyone would advise women like you (or me) that they can function well without serious attention to the best nutritional support they can get.

• Are you implying that everyone ought to take vitamins in the amounts you suggest in Table 5?

No. If you are completely satisfied with your health, your energy level and your mental outlook, and you eat as healthfully as you reasonably can, you very likely do not need supplements. My observation is that young adult men form the largest group in this category. This may explain why some women tell me that their husbands fail to understand the relationship between fatigue, moodiness and nutrition—they simply have never experienced it.

Whether or not to take vitamins should not be an "all or none" decision. For example, those who are reasonably satisfied with their health, energy level and moods may want to take a middle road by supplementing vitamins and minerals at a low level as an "insurance policy." Others who have improved their health through diet and supplements may be able to maintain their good health through excellent diet and perhaps a low level of supplementation. In other words, taking food supplements (or not taking them) should relate to your perceived need, which changes with age, illness, pregnancy, stress level and diet.

There are many good multi-vitamins available through health food shops and other outlets, and in the following sections of this book I mention three by name—Optivite, Procycle, and Magna Natal. One of the reasons that I recommend these is that the full dose for each is at least six tablets per day. This gives the users a great deal of flexibility in finding their own middle ground between high levels of supplements and none at all.

Part II

Overcoming Reproductive System Problems and Challenges

Introduction

As implied in the "Foreword," the main purpose of this book is to offer suggestions on how to assist the natural fertility processes to function normally through proper nutrition. Therefore, Part II may be considered the core of this book. However, three points should be kept in mind as you review the nutritional recommendations that follow.

First, a nutritious diet, as outlined in Part I, is always the highest priority. The *Nutrition Almanac** may be consulted as a reference to identify the best food sources of particular vitamins and minerals. I want to give special emphasis to eating a nutritious diet in case you have turned to this part of the book for an "immediate solution" to some problem without first reading Part I.

Second, in many cases only one or a few micronutrients are mentioned as specifically helpful for a particular condition. While these ones should be stressed, it is my opinion that all others in Table 5 (Chapter 3) should also be taken to prevent imbalances if you choose to supplement. Where a range of dosage is given in Table 5, my suggestion is to try the higher levels of the key nutrients, but use the lower levels for the others.

Finally, I mean it sincerely when I say that the suggestions offered on these pages are not meant to replace the assistance of a medical doctor. Nutrition and medical care are by no means mutually exclusive. A good medical doctor's ability to diagnose, treat and advise is a blessing we are fortunate to have. In my opinion, however, once a diagnosis is made, healing through nutrition should ordinarily be considered the *first* resort. If intervention with drugs or surgery becomes necessary, the importance and value of excellent nutrition is even greater.

* See "Further Reading"

The Normal Fertility-Menstrual Cycle

In this part of the book, we're going to be looking at a number of problems with the female fertility-menstrual cycle. At times this gets rather technical, so you can read this at two different levels. At one level, you can simply note the type of problem and then skip down to the section on "what you can do about it." At the other level, you can read about the research that has sought the causes of the problem and has shown a possible or very definite connection between the problem and certain nutritional deficiencies or dietary and exercise patterns.

In either case, you should have a basic understanding of the normal fertility-menstrual cycle. In that way, you can better understand why certain abnormalities occur when normal functions are disturbed. The process is actually quite complex, but a simplified understanding is sufficient for our purposes. If you would like a more complete description, obtain a copy of *A Physician's Reference to Natural Family Planning* from the Couple to Couple League.*

Normal female fertility requires the proper interaction between several hormones which induce ovulation and maintain the cycle after ovulation. In the early part of the cycle, the pituitary gland secretes follicle stimulating hormone (FSH) which begins the ovulation process by stimulating a follicle (a small sac of cells which contains an ovum) in one of the two ovaries to begin to develop. As the ovarian follicle develops, it secretes estrogen which causes the inner lining of the uterus, the endometrium, to develop. Estrogen also causes the cervix to secrete a mucus discharge which is necessary for normal fertility and sperm migration. (Depending on the quality of the mucus, natural family planning providers refer to it as "less fertile" or "more fertile"; if it is absent the term "dry" is used.) When a certain level of estrogen is reached, the pituitary gland secretes luteinizing hormone (LH) which causes ovulation—that is, the follicle which held the ovum releases it.

* See "Resources"

After ovulation, that same follicle gets a new look and a new name. It becomes yellowish and is therefore called the yellow body or the corpus luteum, and it secretes progesterone which maintains the endometrium for possible implantation. Progesterone also causes the waking (basal) temperature to rise slightly, and the combination of decreased estrogen and increased progesterone causes the cessation of the cervical mucus discharge. After about two weeks, if pregnancy has not occurred, the corpus luteum stops secreting progesterone, and the sudden drop in this hormone causes the inner lining of the uterus to be shed in the process of menstruation. Keep that term, corpus luteum, in mind because it is used frequently in scientific discussion of the fertility cycle. The post-ovulatory part of the cycle is called the luteal phase, and inadequacies in the corpus luteum and the luteal phase are called luteal phase deficiencies.

This understanding of the normal fertility-menstrual cycle is at the heart of natural family planning (NFP). The woman who charts her mucus and temperature signs gains an extremely accurate awareness of where she is in her fertility cycle, and the benefits of this extend beyond family planning. For example, if she is troubled by PMS (which is associated with the luteal phase) she will know from her fertility observations exactly when to expect such symptoms.

If you keep in mind the old slogan, "You are what you eat," you will easily see the possible connection between inadequate nutrition and inadequate functioning of the fertility cycle. The hormones which are so necessary for the normal process are chemicals produced by your body, and they need certain nutrients for their proper production. Furthermore, a certain balance of nutrients is necessary for proper function of the hormones.

It is also necessary to keep in mind that what happens before ovulation can affect the post-ovulatory time of the cycle. For example, if the ovarian follicle fails to develop properly before ovulation, it may also function inadequately after ovulation in the secretion of progesterone. With that brief review, we can look at some of the problems women encounter in their fertility-menstrual cycles and what they can do about them through improved nutrition and/or body balance.

5

Premenstrual Syndrome

In no other reproductive disorder has diet been as strongly implicated as it has been in premenstrual syndrome (PMS), or premenstrual tension (PMT), as it is also called. And in no other reproductive disorder have the nutritional guidelines to improve the condition been so well worked out. The woman who suffers from PMS has every reason to be optimistic that she can help herself to overcome or improve this problem. Because it tends to normalize the levels of the reproductive hormones, the PMS nutritional strategy may also benefit women with infertility, premenopausal symptoms, short luteal phase, and endometriosis.

PMS refers to a large group of symptoms which may occur in women during the post-ovulatory phase of their cycle, though severe PMS may begin earlier and last into the next cycle. Dr. Guy Abraham, the leading American researcher of the nutritional aspects of PMS, has divided the symptoms into four categories as follows:

PMT-A (for anxiety), characterized by nervous tension, mood swings, irritability and anxiety;

PMT-H (for hyperhydration), characterized by weight gain, swelling of extremities, breast tenderness, and abdominal bloating;

PMT-C (for carbohydrate craving), which involves headache, craving for sweets, increased appetite, heart pounding, fatigue, and dizziness or faintness;

PMT-D (for depression), which includes depression, forgetfulness, crying, confusion and insomnia.[1]

Most women who have PMS experience more than one symptom, and symptoms may change from cycle to cycle.

Possible Causes of PMS

Several different causes, all of which relate to dietary and micronutrient imbalances, have been proposed to explain the various forms of PMS.

1) *Abnormal Luteal Function.* Many women with PMS have elevated estrogen levels and low progesterone levels in the luteal phase of their cycles.[2] If **B vitamins** are lacking, the liver cannot inactivate estrogen, and high estrogen levels reduce progesterone levels.[3]

Consumption of animal fats is implicated in PMS because these fats contain arachidonic acid, which is the dietary precursor of a harmful "local hormone," the prostaglandin F_2alpha.[4] This prostaglandin depresses the function of the corpus luteum, which produces the progesterone in the luteal phase.[5]

Conversely, **dietary fiber**, which is simply the indigestible portion of whole plant foods, has the beneficial effect of reducing estrogen levels, apparently by "shielding" estrogens which are excreted in the bile from being reabsorbed into the blood.[6] Women who are free from PMS have been found to eat twice as much dietary fiber as do women who are troubled by this disorder, and while the former consume as much fat, they use mostly vegetable fat, while women with PMS consume mostly animal fat.[7]

Importantly, **vitamin B_6** alone has been shown to elevate progesterone.[8] This vitamin has also significantly reduced the symptoms of PMS in double-blind studies.[9] The entire diet and supplement program developed by Dr. Guy Abraham (presented later) has restored high luteal phase estrogen and

48

low luteal phase progesterone to normal levels while reducing the symptoms of PMS.[10]

2) *Abnormal Fluid Retention*. The hormone aldosterone, which causes the kidneys to retain salt and water, is abnormally elevated in some women with PMS. **Magnesium** deficiency causes excess aldosterone secretion. Both **vitamin B$_6$** and magnesium are necessary for the synthesis of the beneficial chemical, dopamine, which among other functions helps the kidneys to rid the body of salt and water.[11] Intracellular magnesium levels have been found to be lower in women with PMS than in other women.[12] Women with PMS also consume more dairy products than do women without this disorder; besides being a source of animal fat, dairy products, with their unbalanced calcium to magnesium ratio of 10:1, inhibit the absorption of magnesium.[13]

It is extremely useful to realize also that excess sugar consumption causes fluid retention within a day or two of a sugar binge, even when aldosterone levels are normal. And, while excessive salt promotes fluid retention, **adequate salt** prevents over-secretion of aldosterone.[14]

3) *Hypoglycemia*. Low blood glucose levels may contribute to PMS, as the typical hypoglycemic symptoms of faintness, craving for sweets, headache and so forth suggest. Women with PMS consume more sugar and refined carbohydrates than do others.[15] (See Rule 5 in Chapter 1 for an explanation of the relationship between hypoglycemia and sugar consumption.)

A beneficial local hormone, prostaglandin E$_1$, helps to regulate the secretion of insulin, and its deficiency may contribute to PMT-C. This prostaglandin is derived from cis-linoleic acid, which is abundant in **vegetable oils**, especially **safflower oil**. However, for the dietary cis-linoleic acid to be converted to the helpful prostaglandin E$_1$, **magnesium, vitamins B$_3$, B$_6$,** and **C** and **zinc** are all necessary. Saturated fats from animal sources or hydrogenated sources, such as margarine, block this vital conversion; they also favor the synthesis of a harmful antagonistic prostaglandin, the previously mentioned F_2alpha. Decreasing the ratio of calcium to magnesium also decreases the undesirable insulin overresponse to sugar.[16] Abraham's preferred ratio of **calcium to magnesium** is **1:2**, opposite the 2:1 or 3:1 ratio of these two minerals which is usually suggested by nutritional advisors.[17]

Along with sugar, caffeine consumption exacerbates hypoglycemia. **B vitamins** (especially **folic acid**), **potassium** and **chromium** help the body to maintain normal blood glucose levels.

4) *Elevated Levels of the Hormone Prolactin.* Prolactin levels are higher in some women with PMS than in women without this problem.[18] Even men, injected with prolactin in a double-blind study, have reported PMS-like symptoms.[19]

David Horrobin, Ph.D., a highly regarded prolactin researcher, believes that even when prolactin levels appear normal, women with PMS may have a high degree of sensitivity to this hormone. The previously mentioned beneficial prostaglandin E_1 may also help to reduce the effects of prolactin.[20] As noted, adequate dietary **vegetable oil, low saturated fats** and several **vitamins** and **minerals** are all necessary for the body to produce this prostaglandin. These "bottle-necks" in producing E_1 can be bypassed through the use of gamma-linoleic acid, which is found only in human breast milk and in **evening primrose oil.** In three double-blind studies and one open study, this oil in the proprietary form Efamol (up to 4 g/day) was given to women, many with PMS that had been resistant to other treatments. Most improved substantially, especially in the symptoms of depression, irritability, fluid retention and breast discomfort.[21] Evening primrose oil is expensive and therefore is recommended only to those who are not successful with the other nutritional strategies. One to two grams twice daily is an effective intake.[22]

The hypothalamus controls prolactin primarily through inhibition, not stimulation, and prolactin will rise abnormally if it is not properly controlled. Dopamine is the "prolactin-inhibiting factor." **Vitamin B_6** reduces prolactin levels through stimulation of dopamine production.[23] **Magnesium** is also necessary for dopamine synthesis, and so contributes to normal levels of prolactin, along with vitamin B_6. **Zinc** may also suppress prolactin levels.[24] Interestingly, hypoglycemia is a potent stimulus for prolactin release.

5) *Vitamin E Deficiency.* **Vitamin E** (150 to 600 units/day) has been used in a double-blind study to treat PMS. It significantly decreased breast tenderness and the symptoms of PMT-C and PMT-D.[25] Some researchers consider it a mild prostaglandin inhibitor.

6) *Caffeine Consumption.* Even doctors who treat PMS patients largely with pharmacological agents have found that eliminating all of the caffeine sources (coffee, tea, chocolate, cola) is an important first step in managing PMS.[26] These foods are especially implicated in breast cysts and breast pain.[27]

What can you do to alleviate the symptoms of PMS? If you just glance over the preceding paragraphs, you will notice that what you eat or don't eat is implicated in various aspects of PMS. Therefore it makes good sense to look to improved nutrition and diet for your primary attack upon the causes of PMS.

The PMS Diet

Doctor Abraham has formulated a specific nutritional strategy which integrates the foregoing information into practical advice for women with PMS. His dietary guidelines are as follows:

• Limit consumption of refined sugar (5 Tbs/day), salt (3 gram/day), red meat (3 oz/day), alcohol (1 oz/day), coffee, tea and chocolate. [Note: one gram = about 1/30 of 1 ounce of weight.]
• Limit tobacco use.
• Limit intake of protein to 1 gram per kilogram of body weight per day. [1 g per each 2.2 pounds; see below.]
• Rely more on fish, poultry, whole grains and legumes as sources of protein and less on red meat and dairy products.

- Limit intake of dairy products to 2 servings/day.
- Limit intake of fats, mainly saturated and cooked (less than 20% of calories).
- Increase intake of complex carbohydrates (60-70% of calories).
- Increase intake of green leafy vegetables, legumes, whole grains and cereals.
- Increase intake of cis-linoleic-acid-containing foods (safflower oil is an excellent source).[28] [1-2 tablespoons per day of unheated, unrefined oil on your salad; —author's note.]

Protein contents are always given in grams and can be easily found in publications such as the *Nutrition Almanac.** It's helpful to memorize that one cup of milk contains 8 grams of protein, four ounces of meat has about 20, an egg has 6, and a whole wheat peanut butter sandwich has about 10 grams. To estimate your ideal intake, divide your body weight by 2.2, and the result is your ideal intake of protein per day in grams. If you weigh 125 pounds, for example, 125 divided by 2.2 equals 57 grams per day.

PMS Supplements

Doctor Abraham has also formulated a nonprescription multi-vitamin/multi-mineral supplement, Optivite, which is based on his research of the micronutrient needs of women with PMS (see Table 6); it is available at many pharmacies. A very similar supplement, Procycle, may be obtained from Madison Pharmacy Associates in Wisconsin.** Both contain high levels of vitamin B_6 compared to the other B vitamins plus calcium and magnesium in the 1:2 ratio recommended by Abraham. Both are limited in folic acid, which in my opinion should be obtained separately for balance (2,000 mcg/day). Each suggests up to twelve tablets per day, allowing the woman to adjust her dosage as needed. In an open study of Optivite, the best results were obtained among women with PMS when they took six to twelve tablets daily for three or more cycles.[29] In another large study, "one-a-day" vitamins of unspecified potency were useless for PMS, and six tablets per

* See "Further Reading"
** See "Resources"

day of Optivite were more effective than diet modification alone in reducing the symptoms of PMS.[30] Optivite was also effective in the treatment of PMS under double-blind conditions.[31] All of this is solid evidence that dietary supplements in the right dosage can alleviate PMS symptoms.

The general supplement program suggested in Table 5 (Chapter 3) may be used instead, with 200-300 mg of vitamin B_6 and 500-800 mg of magnesium in a 1:1 or 1:2 ratio of calcium to magnesium.

In over 100,000 women who have used Abraham's supplement for several years, no cases of vitamin or mineral toxicity have been reported. Abraham credits this to the balance of the micronutrients within the supplement, as well as his advice *for women to use the lowest effective dose.*[32] Nevertheless, nutritional counseling should be considered for vitamin B_6 supplementation over 200-300 mg per day to avoid toxicity.[33] I do not believe more than this much B_6 is necessary if magnesium, vitamin C and other B vitamins are well supplied. My experience is that women with PMS begin to find relief, often within the first cycle of use, by taking six tablets of Optivite daily (which supplies 300 mg of B_6) along with an additional 500 mg of magnesium. It's not infrequent that one of my natural family planning clients or university students will mention that she's recently tried Optivite and dietary measures and has within a month noticed a definite improvement in both her moods and her energy level.

Certain chemicals may act as vitamin B_6 antagonists and therefore should be avoided whenever possible. These include the hydrazines, which are used in agricultural, pharmaceutical and manufacturing agents. The chemical tartrazine, also called FD&C Yellow No. 5, is a food dye that is converted to hydrazine within the body.[34] According to the late nutritional pioneer Adelle Davis, penicillin, other antibiotics, and many types of drugs may cause a vitamin B_6 deficiency by increasing the need for this vitamin.[35] My own opinion is that antibiotics are the worst vitamin B_6 depletors.

Other aids for the woman with PMS include reasonable body weight, regular exercise, stress reduction and adequate rest. Simply knowing when to expect PMS by using a sympto-thermal chart can be beneficial, and including notes on the type, severity and duration of PMS symptoms is an excellent self-help practice. If the guidelines given here are not helpful within two or three cycles, other causes of PMS-like symptoms, particularly thyroid dysfunction or candidiasis, should be investigated (see Chapter 13, "Candidiasis").

*PMS Access** is a bimonthly newsletter which disseminates self-help information on PMS. It includes a catalogue of useful books and tapes on PMS, and covers all approaches to the management of this condition.

* See "Resources"

Table 6
Optivite (12 tablets)

Vitamins

A	25,000	I.U.
E	200	I.U.
D$_3$ (cholecalciferol)	200	I.U.
Folic acid	400	mcg
B$_1$ (Thiamine)	50	mg
B$_2$ (Riboflavin)	50	mg
B$_3$ (Niacinamide)	50	mg
B$_6$ (Pyroxidine)	600	mg
B$_{12}$	125	mcg
Biotin	125	mcg
Pantothenic acid	50	mg
Choline	625	mg
Inositol	50	mg
Para Amino Benzoic Acid	50	mg
C	3,000	mg
Bioflavinoids	500	mg
Rutin	50	mg

Minerals

calcium	250	mg
magnesium	500	mg
iodine	150	mcg
iron	30	mg
copper	1.0	mg
zinc	50	mg
manganese	20	mg
potassium	95	mg
selenium	200	mcg
chromium	200	mcg

(Adapted from Fuchs, N., M. Hakim, and G. Abraham, M.D., 1985. The effect of a nutritional supplement, Optivite® for Women, on premenstrual tension syndromes: I. Effect on blood chemistry and serum steroid levels during the midluteal phase. J. Appl. Nutr., 37:2-3.)

6

Cycle Irregularities and Female Infertility

A woman's fertility depends upon a complex interaction between several hormones which induce ovulation and maintain the cycle after ovulation. Before proceeding with this section, you may find it helpful to review the brief description of the normal fertility-menstrual cycle which appears at the beginning of Part II (p. 43).

It is also useful to realize that female fertility is not an "all-or-none" phenomenon; rather, a continuum exists between normal high fertility, cycle irregularities, and complete infertility. This is not to imply that irregular cycles generally indicate infertility, although in some women some types of recurring cycle irregularities do signal decreased fertility. Cycle irregularity differs from infertility by a matter of degree, as sprinkles differ from a rainstorm, and therefore the same nutritional guidelines apply to the fertile woman with troublesome cycle characteristics as to the woman having difficulty in conceiving.

The nursing mother, as she gradually makes the transition from complete infertility to normal fertility, illustrates this continuum. Her experience is instructive for non-nursing women with irregular cycles or unexplained infertility.

When the hormones of ovulation, FSH and LH, are consistently low, as in a nursing mother with extended amenorrhea (absence of periods), follicle development does not occur and the endometrium does not develop. The result is that neither ovulation nor menstruation occurs. As she begins to produce more of the reproductive hormones, cervical mucus appears and the endometrium develops. If the nursing mother does not ovulate, eventually the endometrium will be shed anyway, causing spotting or a full, possibly prolonged episode of bleeding. Such a "period" without previous ovulation indicates that an infertile, "anovulatory" cycle has occurred. It is common for a breastfeeding mother to have one or several such anovulatory cycles and periods.

As the inhibition of fertility caused by nursing continues to subside, increased FSH and LH may stimulate an ovarian follicle to develop to some extent, and an immature egg, probably incapable of fertilization, may be ovulated.[1] If so, a basal temperature shift occurs, although it may be less than the usual shift of 4/10ths of one degree Fahrenheit (0.4°F). Since the levels of FSH and LH in the preovulatory stage determine the function of the corpus luteum after ovulation, luteal function may be reduced.[2] A sympto-thermal chart, on which the signs of fertility are recorded, may show this with a luteal (post-ovulatory) phase which is quite a bit shorter than the normal twelve to sixteen days of elevated waking temperatures, and clinical pregnancy (conception plus successful implantation) is less likely if the duration of elevated temperatures in the luteal phase is less than nine to twelve days. Spotting may also occur before the actual period begins while the temperatures are still elevated. Such "irregular shedding" may be yet another manifestation of luteal insufficiency. The entire pattern at this stage of the nursing mother's return to fertility commonly includes an extended patch of "more fertile" mucus prior to ovulation, as well as a delay in ovulation that may cause a long cycle.

Finally, the fertility pattern of the nursing mother returns to its familiar norms, and she may continue to nurse for many months while having fertile ovulatory cycles, or she may conceive again. On the other hand, some women may be unable to become pregnant until after weaning.

Some non-nursing women with apparently normal cycles may still be infertile because of insufficient ovulation-inducing hormones. That is, her mucus, cycle length, thermal shift and luteal phase may all appear normal, but clinical testing reveals that FSH and/or LH levels are insufficient to cause ovulation of a mature egg. The result is either failure to conceive or early miscarriage without development of the tiny conceptus—the newly conceived human life.[3] In such cases induction of ovulation with fertility drugs may enable the woman to overcome her inability to conceive or to carry a pregnancy.

Though the underlying cause is different, this entire pattern, in reverse, is typical of the premenopausal woman as she proceeds from fully fertile cycles to the permanent amenorrhea of the menopause.

Several different factors are responsible for cycle irregularity in either fertile or marginally fertile non-nursing women. In many cases you may never find the precise cause, but you can still take heart from the fact that nutrition by itself can sometimes improve cycle regularity and lead to long-awaited pregnancies. Let's take a look at some of the possible causes of cycle irregularities and female infertility.

Luteal Phase Inadequacy

Inadequate functioning of your fertility hormones can result in these conditions: *short luteal phase, premenstrual spotting, poor thermal shift, extended mucus, scant mucus, amenorrhea, or unexplained infertility.*

In the nursing mother, the hormone prolactin inhibits LH, FSH, and progesterone, and ultimately it contributes to the inadequate luteal phase that is normal for a time in cycling, lactating women. In non-nursing women, elevated prolactin levels are also associated with short luteal phases, amenorrhea, and infertility; "menstrual disorders or infertility may be an early manifestation of prolactin hypersecretion [too much prolactin], with a short luteal phase defect as an early manifestation."[4] The negative effect of elevated prolactin on luteal function and fertility in non-nursing women has been confirmed in other studies as well.[5]

Can nutrition help you to overcome short luteal phase or its related manifestations?

Vitamin B$_6$ alone (200-600 mg/day) has lowered prolactin levels and restored regular cycles to women with the severe overproduction of prolactin which causes both amenorrhea and galactorrhea (milk in the breasts of non-nursing women).[6]

The PMS nutritional program developed by Dr. Guy Abraham contains several elements that reduce prolactin; in reality, it is designed to overcome luteal phase inadequacy which may also contribute to PMS.[7] (See also Chapter 5, particularly "Elevated Levels of the Hormone Prolactin," "The PMS Diet" and "PMS Supplements.") This program of diet and supplements has remarkably restored low luteal phase progesterone and high luteal phase estrogen to normal levels.[8] Women who do not wish to conceive but who show short luteal phases, extended mucus, scant mucus, poor temperature shift or premenstrual spotting may find that the PMS nutritional strategy improves these aspects of their cycles. From a practical standpoint, if such improvement occurs, it will decrease the length of the apparent fertile time (while making the shorter fertile time more fertile) and increase the length of the highly infertile post-ovulatory time. Mucus and temperature patterns have returned to normal within three to six months in some women who have followed Abraham's PMS nutritional plan as well as exercise and stress reduction.[9] With regard to the latter point, adequate rest is an important factor in reducing stress, and one that, along with improved nutrition, should be given a high priority.

In a truly remarkable study, vitamin B$_6$, a critical nutrient for PMS sufferers, was given in 100-800 mg/day doses to fourteen women who had normal menstrual cycles but also had PMS and infertility of eighteen months to seven years' duration. Ten of the fourteen had never borne a child; the other four were experiencing secondary infertility. Twelve of the women conceived, eleven within six months of the B$_6$ therapy! In this study, prolactin levels were not found to change, but progesterone levels were significantly increased in several women, indicating that the vitamin B$_6$ had improved their luteal function.[10]

Barbara Kass-Annese and Dr. Hal Danzer suggest that women with infertility of unknown cause use the entire PMS diet and supplement plan whether or not they have PMS.[11] I suspect that the puzzling "secondary" infertility that occurs in women who have previously conceived with ease may be especially helped by the PMS nutritional strategy because PMS itself is known to become worse after pregnancy, and what is pregnancy if not a nutritional stress?

Low Thyroid Function

When the thyroid gland does not produce enough of its hormones, it results in a condition called hypothyroidism. It can be reflected by or can cause these conditions: *low basal temperatures, unusually long cycles, anovulatory cycles, prolonged "more fertile" mucus, heavy menses or unexplained infertility.*

According to Sheldon S. Stoffer, M.D., a Michigan endocrinologist, menstrual problems may be the first or only symptom of thyroid dysfunction.[12]   Women with pre-ovulatory basal temperatures hovering near 97.2°F. or lower, or with any of the other symptoms listed above, may have on their chart evidence of subclinical thyroid deficiency. (Subclinical means that the thyroid function is not so low as to be considered pathological or to cause a goiter; diagnostic testing, which may be advisable, would probably show it to be in the low range of what is currently accepted as normal.)

What can you do about cycle irregularities which seem to fit the pattern of low thyroid activity?

Adding iodized salt (not plain sea salt) to the diet has improved cycle irregularity and irregular mucus patterns in women who were using little or no iodized salt.[13] If you don't want to consume extra salt, you can get your RDA of **iodine** in almost any kelp tablet. Kelp is a seaweed that grows off some coastal areas and is rich in iodine. Besides iodine, the **B vitamins** and **vitamins C** and **E** aid thyroid function.[14] **Vitamin A**, **zinc** and **selenium** also contribute to thyroid health.[15] Iodine can be toxic at high levels; 150 mcg is the RDA, and Dr. Stuart Berger recommends 1,000 mcg as a maximum.[16] Ocean fish two or three times a week is an excellent source of iodine.

In the mid-eighties a twenty-two-year-old woman who had had two babies in quick succession consulted me about her unusual fertility charts. She had weaned the second baby at six months of age, and when her cycles returned shortly thereafter, her basal temperatures were all well below 97.0°F.—almost a degree lower than normal, and she had experienced four anovulatory cycles in a row. She also had a constant mucus secretion. Since I was a fairly new natural family planning instructor at the time, I telephoned the central office of the Couple to Couple League for further information. They thought it might be hypothyroidism and advised me to recommend that she see a physician about the problem. I relayed this information to her, but I also encouraged her to emphasize iodine and vitamin E in her diet—perhaps to eat more fish. She later reported that she did not eat more fish, but did begin taking a multi-vitamin. It was interesting to see her next chart—the temperatures over a two-week period appeared to "crawl" up onto the chart from their position below it. Shortly afterward she ovulated and resumed normal cycles without needing medical intervention.

Hyperthyroidism

Excessively high thyroid activity is called hyperthyroidism, and it can cause or be reflected in the following conditions: *elevated basal temperatures, scant menses, long cycles, and infertility.*

This problem is the reverse of low thyroid function, but it

can also contribute to cycle irregularity and infertility. However, it is less common than low thyroid function. Aside from the symptoms listed above, hyperthyroidism can cause symptoms unrelated to your fertility-menstrual cycle such as excess sweating, hand tremors, anxiety, elevated resting heart rate and weight loss. Endocrinologist Sheldon Stoffer, M.D., notes that minimal thyroid dysfunction can cause reproductive symptoms, and excess thyroid medication is a possible cause of hyperthyroidism. He treated two women who had been unable to overcome infertility, even after months of care by fertility specialists. Each conceived soon after her thyroid medication [presumably for hypothyroidism] was reduced.[17]

Women who suspect that subclinical hyperthyroidism may be the cause of their cycle irregularities or infertility should first seek accurate medical diagnosis, including measurement of thyroid stimulating hormone (TSH) levels as well as thyroxine levels. They should also carefully investigate the possibility of iodine overdose. Kelp tablets, multi-vitamins, excess iodized salt and ocean fish are sources of iodine that should be considered; the first three should be reduced if iodine consumption exceeds the RDA of 150 mcg. Full-blown hyperthyroidism increases the need for all nutrients because it raises the body's energy expenditure, but nutrition alone cannot improve certain types of hyperthyroidism and medical intervention may be necessary.

Underweight or Too Lean

Being underweight or having too little body fat can cause these conditions: *long cycles, anovulatory cycles, amenorrhea, and infertility.*

Both your ratio of weight to height and your ratio of fat to muscle affect your fertility-menstrual cycles for several reasons. First of all, fatty tissue is a storehouse for the sex hormones, and it converts androgens (male hormones) to estrogen, which provides one-third of the total estrogen in normal, premenopausal women.[18] Second, lean women also have higher than average amounts of a protein which binds estrogen; therefore, they have less free estrogen.[19] Third, in underweight or excessively lean women the hypothalamus, which is the part of the brain that controls the pituitary gland, does not properly stimulate the fertility hormones, FSH and LH.[20] For these and perhaps other reasons, being underweight or having too little body fat can have adverse effects upon your cycles.

The extreme dieting of anorexia nervosa, the self-starvation disorder, causes anovulatory cycles and loss of menstruation. When the ratio of body fat to muscle drops only slightly below a critical percentage, the fertility cycle can be affected. In fact, gaining or losing just three pounds can tip the balance toward cycling or amenorrhea.[21] In one study, seventeen of twenty-six underweight women who had been infertile for more than four years conceived after they gained an average of eight pounds each.[22]

What is sometimes overlooked, though, even by medical doctors, is that women of supposedly "ideal" weight, or even somewhat higher than "ideal" weight, may experience loss of menses or greatly delayed ovulation because they, too, are underweight! I have personally counseled several women with total amenorrhea for months after seemingly sensible weight loss. These women were emphatically not overdieting. Yet regaining just a few pounds restored the cycle. For example, a young woman who had previously conceived easily consulted me after her physician could offer no explanation for her prolonged amenorrhea. The amenorrhea coincided with her loss of forty pounds through dieting, and she was maintaining her "ideal" weight. I advised her to regain just a few of the lost pounds. In less than three months, when she had regained seven pounds, she conceived the child for whom she had been hoping.

I have seen enough very long cycles and complete amenorrhea caused by dieting to state emphatically: "Ideal" weight, by American standards, may be too low for fertility in some women. Gaining just three or five pounds can restore fertility or regular cycles. Any woman who is thin or average or who is dieting should consider carrying a few more pounds if long cycles or amenorrhea are a problem. Women with secondary infertility should attempt to restore themselves to the body build—weight and fat to muscle ratio—at which they conceived previously.

Note well that women who exercise vigorously (runners, gymnasts, swimmers, ballet dancers, body builders) are converting body mass from fat to muscle, and they may also experience delayed ovulation or complete infertility and amenorrhea when their total body fat drops below the critical level of around twenty percent.[23] I have seen this occur even when body weight has been completely normal. What this means is that a woman needs sufficient weight for her height and a sufficient ratio of fat to muscle in order to have normal fertility-menstrual cycles.

What can you do if you are experiencing menstrual cycle "irregularities" that may be related to being underweight or being too trim?
Review the first part of this book and make sure you start eating enough good foods to achieve the proper weight for your height. If you are the right weight but have been exercising vigorously, cut back on your exercise, and let some of your normal body fat return; or add a few pounds to your "ideal" weight. If you have an eating disorder such as anorexia or bulimia, you should get competent medical or psychological help.

In my opinion, women with very long cycles, anovulatory cycles or amenorrhea should never undergo medically induced ovulation (Clomid, Pergonal) until they have thoroughly tried to improve their fertility through proper body build (weight/height and fat/muscle ratios) and improved nutrition.

Overweight

Being overweight can cause *cycle irregularity, amenorrhea, or infertility even with regular cycles.*
The role of body fat in female fertility is an essential one,

as the preceding section illustrates. Fat is a metabolically active tissue, and among other functions it converts circulating androgens ("male" hormones) to estrogen. Too much body fat, though, contributes to elevated levels of estrogen,[24] which decreases corpus luteal function.[25] It may be for these reasons that obesity is well known to cause infertility in some women.

Nevertheless, I have seen this important factor overlooked or discounted by physicians treating obese women who were experiencing difficulty in conceiving. For example, I counseled an obese woman who had complicating factors in her infertility that made induction of ovulation with fertility drugs an apparent necessity. She had had three previous pregnancies, and had had at least twelve months of induced cycles before conceiving each time. Her physicians had never informed her of the effect of obesity on fertility. When she consulted me before her fourth pregnancy, I suggested that she lose a moderate amount of weight (she was probably seventy pounds overweight). Four months and forty pounds later, she conceived during the first induced cycle. She stated that she believed that the weight loss had made the difference. In another instance, an obese woman had repeatedly undergone induction of ovulation without achieving pregnancy. Her doctor had told her that he would induce her to ovulate until she lost weight, implying to her that treatment with fertility drugs could overcome the effects of her obesity.

If you are quite overweight and are experiencing cycle irregularity or infertility even with regular cycles, where should you start?

I do not believe that induction of ovulation can necessarily substitute for weight loss when an overweight woman is experiencing infertility. Certainly the obvious problem of overweight should be dealt with before such intervention with drugs is considered. Moderately overweight women with irregular cycles or mucus problems or with unexplained infertility should also attempt to approach their ideal weight a bit more closely. The overweight woman should be careful to lose weight slowly with wholesome nutrition and regular exercise. She should attempt to overcome hypoglycemia with small, frequent snacks of good food, avoidance of caffeine and sugar (see Rule 5, Chapter 1), and appropriate supplements (see Table 5 in Chapter 3 as well as the discussion of hypoglycemia in Chapter 5). She should not despair of losing all the weight necessary to attain her "ideal" weight but should just set a modest goal such as twenty pounds. Finally, she and her husband should not overlook less obvious factors that may also contribute to her cycle irregularity or their infertility.

Discontinuing Birth Control Pills

Discontinuing birth control pills may have several effects on the fertility-menstrual cycle: *heavy menses, constant less fertile mucus, and delayed ovulation.*

The birth control pill, like any synthetic drug taken for a prolonged period of time, depletes certain vitamins. **Folic acid, vitamins B_2, B_6, B_{12},** and **C** are particularly mentioned as being adversely affected by the Pill.[26] All of these should be emphasized. **Vitamin A** levels may drop after discontinuing the Pill,[27] and perhaps 10,000 to 20,000 I.U. of vitamin A will help eliminate the heavy menses that may result from low levels of this vitamin. (See also Chapter 7, "Difficult Menstruation.") **Vitamin E** and **selenium** may help to restore the ovaries to proper function also. If depression, irritability or lack of sexual desire have been problems during use of oral contraceptives, the PMS nutritional strategy is the best bet to reverse these common side effects of the Pill (see Chapter 5, especially "The PMS Diet" and "PMS Supplements"). The Pill has been strongly associated with yeast overgrowth, and ex-Pill users who are experiencing prolonged reproductive problems or general poor health may wish to obtain more information about this newly discovered and still controversial disorder (see Chapter 13, "Candidiasis").

What can you do to alleviate the residual effects of the Pill if you are discontinuing it?

It seems to me that the sensible thing to do would be to double-check your regular diet with the recommendations in Part I; if you have any of the above effects (or other cycle irregularities), consider using supplements as suggested above. My strong opinion is that women coming off the Pill must make extra nutritional efforts to overcome its known deleterious effects, and you will do yourself a special favor to consult with someone who is qualified to counsel you about diet and supplements.

Caffeine Consumption

Coffee and other sources of caffeine can cause *cycle irregularity and even infertility in some women.*

The relationship between caffeine consumption and decreased fertility was strictly anecdotal until the late eighties when the effects of caffeine on achieving pregnancy were investigated. In a 1988 study, women who used more than the equivalent of one cup of coffee per day took significantly longer to conceive than did those who used less, and high caffeine users experienced longer delays in conceiving than did lower level users.[28] This finding was quickly confirmed by other researchers who studied a large number of women.[29]

Not long before these studies were published, a woman experiencing secondary infertility of about eighteen months asked me about her problem. I suggested that she cut out sugar and caffeine, eat nutritiously, and try to drop a few pounds, as she was rather overweight. She conceived two months later, and reported that the only change she had made was to reduce her coffee consumption from six or seven mugs per day to one or one and a half cups daily. She also reported that in the year previous to conception, her cycles had become longer and longer, causing her, a non-NFP user, the inconvenience of repeated pregnancy testing.

Could this be you?

If you are astounded that one can consume so much coffee, you are probably not a caffeine "addict"; if you didn't bat an eye, perhaps you should cut down on your caffeine! This is true even if you aren't presently experiencing any direct adverse effects.

I believe that heavy caffeine users are attempting to overcome hypoglycemia (see Chapter 1, Rule 5 and the discussion of hypoglycemia in Chapter 5). Emphasis on the **B vitamins**, especially **folic acid** (perhaps 2,000 mg/day), small, frequent meals high in complex carbohydrates, and strict limiting of sweet treats are great helps in overcoming low blood glucose. I truly believe that anyone experiencing cycle irregularity or any type of infertility should reduce caffeine-containing foods, drugs and beverages to the equivalent of one to two cups of coffee per *week*.

Sensitivity to Night Lighting

Unlikely as it sounds, sensitivity to night lighting may cause *scant or patchy mucus, prolonged more fertile mucus, short luteal phases, other cycle irregularities, and infertility even with regular cycles.*

As anyone who has ever suffered jet lag can attest to, the body has a definite "biological clock" that resists resetting. This rhythm is entrained by the natural day-night cycle, and nerve impulses that originate from the light receptors of the eyes ultimately affect many of the body's hormones, including the reproductive hormones. The effects of light and dark on reproductive capability are very apparent and well studied in reptiles, birds, and mammals; in them it involves the pineal gland which directly or indirectly responds to the light-dark rhythm. Such influences are less apparent and are poorly understood in humans. This may be so because the natural day-night cycle is disrupted by our modern electric lights, but people in other parts of the world are more aware of this relationship. For example, my husband and I taught NFP to a couple from Africa who told us that their native expression for menstruation is to be "in the moon." Theirs is a very pro-child culture, and the wife told us that her mother advised her to have intercourse during the dark phase of the moon in order to conceive, as their cycles follow the lunar cycles. It is also known clinically that blind girls enter puberty sooner than sighted girls, an effect believed to be mediated through the pineal gland.

Joy DeFelice, R.N., Director of Natural Family Planning Classes at Sacred Heart Medical Center, Spokane, Washington, has since 1976 studied the effect of artificial night illumination on the menstrual cycle and fertility in women NFP users. Her observations are as simple as they are striking—eliminating light from the sleeping quarters can improve mucus patterns and cycle irregularities, and has ended infertility in many cases.[30] Women who have carefully reduced night lighting in their bedrooms typically experience improvement in their mucus or temperature patterns within one to three cycles, and pregnancy among couples previously experiencing infertility has been achieved in an average of five cycles.[31]

Lest you wonder how small amounts of light can affect a sleeping woman, realize that light rays are quite capable of penetrating the eyelids, and the dark-adapted retina is exquisitely sensitive even to very low level illumination. A specific neural route from the eyes sends information about lighting to the pineal gland; this gland responds to light-related neural stimuli by secreting or failing to secrete several hormones which in animals, at least, markedly affect reproduction.

For most women, the sources of night illumination in the bedroom are easily identified and controlled—hall lights, digital clocks, street lights and so forth. Some women may even need to rid their room of light from the crack under the door, from electric blanket controls, or from moonlight filtering through lightweight window blinds. A few women who do not show improved menstrual cycles after three to four cycles of night darkness may respond to a regimen of reduced night lighting, except for three nights of low to moderate illumination (mimicking moonlight) beginning two days after more fertile mucus is seen.[32] An irregular bedtime does not seem to be a factor in this phenomenon provided the woman receives sufficient hours of darkness, and Mrs. DeFelice advises night workers to sleep in a darkened room during the day.[33]

However, for those who have recently discontinued birth control pills, who have experienced a miscarriage, who are ending the natural infertility of breastfeeding or who are bottlefeeding a baby, she does not recommend the regimen of three nights with lighting but only the constant night darkness. In these circumstances, the cycles should be allowed to "settle down" on their own for a few months.[34] Night darkness can also improve the ambiguous mucus of the breastfeeding or bottlefeeding mother, as well as heavy bleeding, prolonged bleeding or constant spotting.[35] Mrs. DeFelice has also linked night illumination to early miscarriage in many cases.[36]

Is there a link between such excessive sensitivity to night lighting and nutrition? I don't know the answer to that, but I would like to offer some strictly speculative ideas. If one compares the reproductive symptoms of nocturnal light sensitivity as listed by Mrs. DeFelice to the symptoms of luteal phase inadequacy already described under the heading with that name, one cannot fail to notice their similarities. Short luteal phases, scant or extended mucus, and even early miscarriage are associated with both. According to Dr. Guy Abraham, PMS can be another manifestation of luteal phase inadequacy. He links deficiency of B vitamins and magnesium to this condition, as well as excessive animal fat consumption and inadequate intake of fiber and unsaturated vegetable oils.[37]

This speculation may be taken a bit further. Dr. Abraham postulates that B vitamin deficiency and magnesium deficiency lead to elevated levels of the brain chemical serotonin, which in turn contribute to the disturbances of PMS.[38] Control of pituitary hormone secretions involves appropriate levels of serotonin as well as other brain chemicals such as dopamine, and it is noteworthy that serotonin stimulates prolactin secretion.[39] Serotonin is produced abundantly by the pineal gland, but only in the light; its output drops off markedly in the dark.[40] If serotonin levels are already excessive due to vitamin or mineral deficiency, does even a bit of lighting in the bedroom cause enough additional serotonin to be synthesized to disrupt the pituitary hormones and thus the menstrual cycle? Is the cycle disruption caused by the stimulatory effect of serotonin on prolactin? Perhaps extreme darkness enables a woman with excess serotonin production to compensate by reducing such serotonin production at night.

What nutrients might benefit a woman who seems to require constant night darkness to have regular cycles? Dopamine reduces serotonin, and the previously mentioned vitamin B_6 and magnesium are necessary for dopamine synthesis.[41] The dietary precursor of serotonin is the amino acid tryptophan which is abundant in milk products. Interestingly, Dr. Abraham recommends that milk products be limited in those who have PMS.

In the less common situation in which several nights of light in the bedroom are necessary to promote cycle regularity or fertility, it may be that higher levels of serotonin are beneficial for such individuals at midcycle. Perhaps a bedtime glass of milk would be beneficial during the midcycle time when night lighting is recommended.

It may be worth noting that deficiency of the B vitamin riboflavin (B_2) causes excessive sensitivity to bright lighting. Whether or not this may be involved in nocturnal sensitivity which affects the menstrual cycle, I do not know, but all the B vitamins generally are involved in similar enzyme systems.

What can you do if sensitivity to night lighting could be your situation?

If you want to pursue the possible nutrition connection indicated above, you should get good nutritional counseling and should consider Dr. Abraham's PMS strategy (see Chapter 5, particularly "The PMS Diet" and "PMS Supplements"). It will, of course, take a bit of effort in some cases to eliminate night light, perhaps some opaque window shades and curtains. If all else fails, you might try to obtain more information on this fascinating topic by writing to Mrs. Joy DeFelice.*

* See "Resources"

Other Causes of Poor Mucus Patterns, Cycle Irregularities or Infertility

The experience of the Couple to Couple League is that **vitamin A** helps to restore mucus to the "classic" pattern, especially when the problem is a lack of the more fertile mucus. A well-chewed carrot daily might be sufficient, or 10,000 to 20,000 I.U. per day is an adequate supplement. Vitamin A excess, however, can cause scanty menses or amenorrhea.[42] So can extremely excessive dietary carotene (the vitamin A precursor found in yellow and green vegetables), or carotene from "tanning" pills.[43] **Zinc** and **vitamin E** increase the effectiveness of vitamin A.

Over-the-counter cold and allergy remedies which reduce respiratory mucus can also reduce cervical mucus. Conversely, the guaifenesin in many expectorant cough syrups may increase the fluidity of cervical mucus. Vitamin C, the B vitamin pantothenic acid, the amino acid histidine, and the bioflavinoids (considered by some to be true vitamins) are better solutions to hay fever and cold symptoms than are drugs. Bioflavinoids are found in the white membranes of citrus fruits or are available as supplements. Sucking on zinc lozenges may help prevent the cold in the first place.

Vaginal infections also disrupt mucus secretion, interfering with observation of mucus. Chapter 8, "Vaginal Infections," may be of value to women concerned about this problem.

Endometriosis, which is one source of pain during menstruation, can also cause infertility. It is discussed in Chapter 7, "Difficult Menstruation."

Yeast overgrowth, or candidiasis, has been implicated in several disorders of the male and female reproductive systems. Cycle irregularity and infertility have both been attributed to candidiasis by the growing minority of medical doctors who recognize this disease. See Chapter 13, "Candidiasis" for further information on this topic.

Other Notes on Infertility

Nutrition alone can affect fertility, as some of the clinical studies demonstrate. Let me close, however, with an anecdote which illustrates a wider context.

Charlene A. of Fort Wayne, Indiana, conceived with ease three times in her twenties (miscarrying between the births of two daughters). Thereafter, however, she was unable to become pregnant. When she was thirty-eight, a doctor told her and her husband that there was "nothing wrong" but that she was too old to pursue treatment. At age forty-one, after fourteen years of infertility, she and I met when she enrolled in my university class in human anatomy and physiology. I was pregnant at the time, and more than once she commented to me about her yearning for another child and her long-standing infertility despite regular cycles. I sensed her lack of peace and suggested that she and her husband take our Couple to Couple League class (which they eventually did).

Meanwhile, she constantly complained about the difficulty of my class, and to talk her out of dropping it, I suggested she drop caffeine and sugar instead. (I've suggested this to many overstressed students over the years, with pretty fair success.) She took this advice to heart, and each week thereafter, when the class met, she raved to me about the difference nutrition made: "I feel so much better ... I've lost ten pounds without even trying... I'd never go back to sugar ... I've even talked my husband into good nutrition." The two of them soon enrolled in an excellent fitness course emphasizing sound nutrition and moderate exercise. Two months later, to her absolute astonishment and joy, she realized that she was pregnant. I will never forget her incredible joy—the morning of the final exam—as she exclaimed again and again, "It's a miracle!"

You probably expect that the end of this story is a baby, but if so you are only half right. She had a healthy daughter the following August, and shortly afterward enrolled in our natural family planning course. When the baby was thirteen months old, she weaned in order to conceive again. Doubting her ability to do so naturally, she sought the services of her obstetrician. After four months of inducing her to ovulate with fertility drugs, he dismissed her somewhat rudely: "You're never going to get pregnant." Six months later, using a combination of charting, timing, maintenance of the weight at which she had previously conceived, ideal diet and supplements similar to those in Table 5 (Chapter 3), she did conceive! She had the healthiest pregnancy and birth of any woman I have ever met; her lovely daughter, her fourth, was born when she was forty-three.

This, my favorite anecdote, illustrates several things that may have been helpful—good diet, supplements, attention to weight, and timing of intercourse (at least the second time around). Other points are also important to mention: the simultaneous improvement of both spouses' diets; a positive attitude despite the clear ticking of the "biological clock" and the discouragement of doctors who would not or could not help; and the willingness to continue self-help techniques during and after unsuccessful medical intervention. Last but not least was bringing the infertility in prayer before the Lord.

I'm sure that Charlene would not recommend that you experience fourteen years of infertility before you try nutrition, and it is useful to realize that the large majority of normally fertile couples who have noncontraceptive intercourse regularly (say twice a week) will conceive within six months. If conception has not occurred by then, timing of intercourse, excellent nutrition, sleeping room light reduction, and the other fertility strategies taught by the Couple to Couple League* should all be implemented by both husband and wife. If in six or nine months conception has still not occurred, by all means continue with the nutrition, timing, and so forth, but seek the assistance of an infertility specialist. I cannot recommend strongly enough that you find a specialist who deals primarily with infertility, even if you must go to a larger town to do so. It has been my experience again and again, through our infertility clients, that the obstetrician-gynecologist who *also* happens to treat infertility is sometimes

* See "Resources"

an inadequate choice for the couple having difficulty in achieving pregnancy. The specialist who works with infertility on a daily basis can bring a systematic, comprehensive approach to diagnosing and treating infertility that contrasts sharply with the more limited approach of the obstetrician-gynecologist who deals with this problem only sporadically.

Finally, I take issue with that usually unsolicited advice to infertile couples, "Relax!" Emotional or physical stress can cause a temporary delay in ovulation, but this does not interfere with the ability to conceive in that cycle when ovulation finally occurs. Unless you are under extremely prolonged, extremely severe stress, you should look elsewhere to explain infertility.

Please, if you are not infertile, don't suggest that your infertile friends relax. I have never spoken to a woman anxious to conceive who was not hurt and worried by that counterproductive advice. I facetiously encourage our infertility clients to "go ahead and be uptight"—knowing that it doesn't matter is good for their peace of mind!

7

Difficult Menstruation

The typical menstrual period lasts about five days, with two or three days of moderate bleeding followed by two or three days of light flow. Some women, however, consistently experience heavy or prolonged menstrual flows, sometimes up to nine or ten days. Other women experience very painful menstruation, sometimes to the point of being bedridden. Such menses are not normal, and my experience is that nutrition can be a powerful tool in overcoming these difficulties.

Heavy or Prolonged Menstruation

"Heavy menstruation" (menorrhagia) refers to excessive blood loss; by "prolonged menses" I refer to menstruation that lasts more than six or seven days. At the beginning of what will be a long cycle (for example, forty days) a woman may experience a longer, heavier period than when her cycle will be shorter. This is so because the hormones that stimulate ovulation contribute to building up the endometrium, and these hormones appear earlier in shorter cycles and later if that cycle will be a long one.

What can you do if you are troubled by unusually heavy or long periods?

If you have long cycles, you might get help by attempting

to shorten your cycle length. Low thyroid function may be the underlying cause of both heavy menses and long cycles. If so, review "Low Thyroid Function" in Chapter 6. If cycle lengths are normal, emphasis on the general principles of good nutrition as outlined in Part I may make a difference by providing the body with the nutrients needed to improve hormonal levels or to aid the clotting process. If nutritional aids do not alleviate the heavy or prolonged menstruation, medical diagnosis should be sought.

Vitamin A deficiency has been documented in women with heavy menstruation. In one study, supplements of 60,000 I.U. of vitamin A to women with menorrhagia markedly reduced or completely eliminated the problem within a month.[1] *While this is too much vitamin A for one to take without the guidance of a knowledgeable physician*, supplementing 20,000 I.U. on a daily basis is considered safe.[2] **Beta carotene**, the vitamin A precursor found abundantly in the yellow and dark green vegetables, has less potential for toxicity, and such vegetables as carrots, sweet potatoes, squash and spinach should be emphasized. **Zinc** and **vitamin E** assist with vitamin A metabolism, and E in particular contributes to normal menstrual flow.[3]

At one of our natural family planning classes, a woman showed me a chart with eight days of menses during a cycle of only twenty-five days. I alerted her to the value of vitamin A in such cases, as women with short cycles normally have short duration of menses. At the very next meeting, a month later, this young woman showed me her most recent chart, with only a five-day period. She had tried vitamin A supplements (5,000 I.U./day), and she said that this was the first cycle within her recent memory with bleeding of less than eight days.

Elevated levels of vitamin A which are caused by oral contraceptive use contribute to the scanty bleeding sometimes seen in birth control pill users. Conversely, discontinuing the Pill lowers vitamin A, which may contribute to post-Pill menorrhagia.[4]

Efficient blood clotting is essential to normal menstrual

flow. **Vitamin K** is involved in the production of several clotting proteins. It is frequently assumed to be plentiful in the body since "friendly" bacteria within the large intestine synthesize it, and it is available in the diet if dark green leafy vegetables and the cole crops are eaten. However, antibiotics and chlorinated water harm the intestinal bacteria, and typical Americans eat far too little of the vitamin K-rich foods. Emphasis on these foods and regular intake of bacteria-containing **yogurt** or **acidophilus** tablets will help provide vitamin K, especially if nonessential antibiotics and aspirin, which depletes this vitamin, are avoided.

The **bioflavinoids**, found abundantly in the white rind and sectional membranes of citrus fruits, strengthen capillary walls and therefore are useful to moderate the tendency to heavy bleeding. They are also available as supplements.

Calcium is required at several stages of the clotting mechanism; **vitamin D** is required for calcium absorption. Adequate **magnesium** also helps the body to use calcium. Calcium deficiency stemming from milk allergy or poor diet may underlie some cases of menorrhagia.

Chlorophyll seems to enhance blood clotting; the tablets or liquid which are available at better health food stores may be taken shortly before and during menstruation (60 mg/day or that amount after each meal as needed). There is no need to supplement chlorophyll all month; the effect occurs within a short time of taking it. Chlorophyll also rapidly controls postpartum bleeding, according to midwives familiar with its use. Like chlorophyll, **cayenne pepper tablets** (also called **capsicum**) quickly slow any type of bleeding. Using both together is particularly effective.

Heavy, prolonged bleeding which is due to hormonal imbalance is often treated with synthetic progesterone (Provera) or birth control pills. The following anecdote illustrates how appropriate medical intervention and nutritional counseling may have enabled a young girl with severe menorrhagia to avoid these powerful steroid hormones. Only twelve years old, this girl lost half her blood volume during a heavy, prolonged period of which her parents were at first unaware.

When they realized it, her hemoglobin was an extremely anemic 6.5—normal is 13 or better—and she was still bleeding. The attending gynecologist prescribed Provera, but what little of it she did not vomit did no good. At the parents' request, a transfusion of relatives' blood was arranged. It did not stop the bleeding, but it did bring her hemoglobin to an improved though still anemic 10. The gynecologist warned the parents that because of the severity of the situation, birth control pills were the probable next step, but he was willing to take a "wait-and-see" attitude for a short while. The parents, well aware of the side effects of the Pill, turned to nutritional counseling. Cayenne pepper tablets (520 mg 5 times daily) helped slow the bleeding significantly. The girl also began taking an excellent nonprescription multi-vitamin/multi-mineral, Magna Natal by Radiance,* which supplies 10,000 I.U. of vitamin A, 75 mg/mcg of the B vitamins, 60 mg of iron and generous amounts of the other micronutrients. The goal was two-fold: to enable her body to produce more of its own hormones and to overcome the anemia. Her next period was very heavy but manageable; two months later, she was no longer anemic and had a normal menses. Nine months later, her mother reported that she still tended toward heavy periods but was "definitely helped" by the cayenne pepper during her menses. Aside from the transfusion, her mother credits her daughter's faithfulness in taking the vitamins, the cayenne pepper, and plenty of rest as the factors that enabled the girl to recover rapidly from this frightening incident.

If menorrhagia has been severe enough to cause anemia, as in the above anecdote, do not make the mistake of supplementing only iron to overcome it. Iron supplements can be toxic, in fact, and should be used sparingly.[5] The B vitamins, including **folic acid, B$_6$**, and **B$_{12}$, vitamins C** and **E, copper** and adequate **protein** are among the nutrients which are also necessary to produce new red blood cells. Good foods for overcoming anemia are liver, spinach, brewer's yeast, and citrus fruits.

See "Resources"

Painful Menses

Pain is a symptom, severe pain the more so. Menstrual cramps and pain may simply reflect common Western dietary imbalances, or they may be a sign of endometriosis, uterine tumors, infection or other abnormalities. Diagnosis is essential if menstrual pain is worse than the moderate discomfort that is so common, especially among younger women who have never borne children.

The causes of simple dysmenorrhea (painful menstrual periods) and PMS are not the same, yet both share one common aspect. Elevated levels of certain prostaglandins are known to be involved in menstrual pain and cramps,[6] and the same prostaglandins also contribute to the deficient luteal phase of PMS.[7] The PMS nutritional plan, among other things, is designed to reduce synthesis of these harmful prostaglandins. For this reason, the PMS nutritional strategy may be helpful for dysmenorrhea (see "The PMS Diet" and "PMS Supplements" in Chapter 5.) Substantial supplements of **magnesium** (800-1,000 mg/day) may also help reduce uterine cramping, assuming calcium and vitamin D are adequate. Magnesium has relieved severe menstrual cramps in teenage girls, even in cases where codeine has failed.[8]

The "nonsteroid anti-inflammatory drugs" (aspirin, ibuprofen [Advil, Motrin]) are indeed effective in reducing menstrual discomfort; they do so by blocking the production of the previously mentioned harmful prostaglandins. Why not use them? There is a sound reason to avoid them; according to an outstanding prostaglandin researcher, they may exacerbate PMS by blocking the production of a "helpful" prostaglandin.[9]

Endometriosis can cause very severe pain during menstruation, pain during intercourse, and heavy or irregular bleeding. It has become common among modern Western women who experience cycle after cycle uninterrupted by pregnancy and breastfeeding. This disease begins when endometrial tissue moves backward through the fallopian tubes during the menses and is deposited within the abdominal cavity. Living cells in this tissue can proliferate within the abdomen, and when these abnormal "implants" are stimulated by cyclic hormonal changes, they build up and then bleed, causing the intense pain. Scarring and inflammation from the endometrial implants results in infertility in about one-third of women who have the disease. While the factors that ultimately cause endometriosis are not well understood, some researchers believe that hormonal imbalance or immune system deficiency may promote the abnormal growths.[10]

Can you alleviate the symptoms of endometriosis through nutrition?

Worth considering is a possible link between PMS and endometriosis. Doctors Joel Hargrove and Guy Abraham found that half of 137 PMS patients who underwent exploratory surgery for menstrual pain or other problems had endometriosis. These researchers believe that "the underlying pathophysiology in both conditions [PMS and endometriosis] may be abnormal luteal function."[11]

Doctor Hargrove, who is director of a PMS clinic in Vanderbilt, Tennessee, reports that 80 to 90 percent of women with endometriosis also have PMS. He has found that **vitamin B$_6$**, which is a key vitamin for nutritional management of PMS, is also useful for symptomatic self-help treatment of endometriosis. He cautions that the daily dosage should not exceed 500 mg, nor should this amount be taken throughout the entire month.[12] Other physicians recommend that women with endometriosis implement the complete PMS nutritional strategy developed by Dr. Guy Abraham.[13]

This diet and supplement program has been consistently shown to improve luteal function by decreasing estrogen and increasing progesterone levels.[14] Progesterone secreted by the corpus luteum prevents contractions of the uterus, which may be one link between luteal function and endometriosis. While I am aware of no study in which the PMS nutritional plan has overcome infertility specifically related to endometriosis, the woman experiencing difficulty in conceiving because of this disease would be well advised to implement the PMS program vigorously. It seems to me that this nutritional plan could possibly help prevent recurrence of the disease following laser surgery to remove the abnormal endometrial tissue.

You may contact the Endometriosis Association* for further information on all aspects of this disorder.

The diet and supplements suggested here phenomenally helped a twenty-four-year-old single woman with the worst dysmenorrhea I have ever encountered. Her concerned older sister asked if she could bring her sister to me to discuss this problem. During our visit she described abdominal and back pain so wrenching she could hardly walk; she would be so ill that she spent three to five days in bed each month. I suggested that she consider Dr. Abraham's diet and nutritional supplements as in Table 5 (Chapter 3), including about 1,000 mg magnesium in a 2:1 ratio to calcium. She took the list of supplements and selected her own brands of vitamins from a health food shop. She felt "a thousand percent" better during her next period, and by the third cycle was "five thousand percent" better. Her sister and I chatted ten months later; she reported that the younger woman no longer misses any work, her PMS has also improved, and she is "five thousand percent better—at least!"

See "Resources"

8

Vaginal Infections

Occasionally in my counseling as a natural family planning instructor, a woman will ask if an unusual vaginal discharge is "just mucus" or is an infection. Other times the caller will be quite sure she has an infection but is interested in knowing more about self-help techniques for overcoming it or preventing future occurrences.

Among those who have no reason to be concerned about sexually transmitted diseases, there are only two major types of vaginal infections—yeast, and the less common bacterial infections. Both are better prevented than cured so even those who have never had either may want to read this section. Since both have been related to various kinds of artificial birth control, the exclusive use of natural family planning for child spacing in itself is a major preventive of these annoying, uncomfortable infections. In addition, the woman who practices modern NFP is aware of the ordinary, healthy cervical mucus discharge and thus has the benefit of early recognition should infection occur.

Yeast Infections

These all-too-common infections may be identified by "itching, caked discharge that smells like baking bread, and reddening of the labia and sometimes the upper thighs."[1] The common yeast *Candida albicans* normally inhabits the healthy vagina, but the decreased acidity and increased synthesis of glycogen (a natural carbohydrate) that occur during pregnancy or use of oral contraceptives favor proliferation and infection. Intrauterine devices (IUDs) and contraceptive sponges also encourage yeast.[2] Antibiotics contribute importantly to yeast infections by destroying the "friendly" bacteria that inhabit the vagina and naturally inhibit yeast organisms. Since yeast thrives on sugar, overconsumption of the simple carbohydrates, including fruit juices, stimulates their growth. Irritations in or around the vagina can also trigger outbreaks of yeast:

Tight, insulating clothing... feminine hygiene sprays, deodorant toilet paper, and commercial douches may irritate vaginal tissues and predispose women to yeast infections .... Tampons, especially the superabsorbant variety, may dry and irritate the vagina.[3]

What can you do to prevent yeast infections or to fight them if they are already a problem?

Avoiding the causes given above, when possible, is the best preventive. If antibiotics are truly necessary, **yogurt** eaten daily during and following treatment will help restore normal intestinal bacteria. More effective than yogurt are capsules containing **acidophilus**, or "friendly" bacteria, which may be obtained from health food shops and taken with each meal. **Vitamin A** generally aids the health of all of the body's mucous membranes, and **vitamin B$_6$** and **magnesium** are particularly deficient in individuals with *Candida* problems.[4]

With reference to the role of sugar, one hundred women with chronic vaginal yeast infections were found to have

... excessive oral ingestion of dairy products, artificial sweeteners and sucrose [table sugar]. Eliminating excessive use of these foods brought about a dramatic reduction in the incidence and severity of *Candida* vulvovaginitis.[5]

One of our Couple to Couple League clients ended twenty years of treatment for chronic yeast infections by limiting sugar and caffeine and taking supplements similar to those in Table 5 (Chapter 3). She has not had a recurrence in three years.

A commonly recommended self-treatment for minor yeast infections is douching with plain yogurt, either undiluted or diluted enough for ease of flow. Dr. John Trowbridge includes complete directions for a yogurt douche in his book, *The Yeast Syndrome.** He suggests use of a 60 ml irrigating syringe, a lying-down position while douching, subsequent rinsing externally but not internally, and use of sanitary napkins to prevent leakage.[6] Normally, I am completely opposed to douching because it abnormally alters the vaginal environment. However, the Trowbridge sort of douche for the purpose of preventing yeast infection during antibiotic treatment or to overcome infection would be an exception.

Intercourse should be avoided if yeast infection is present in order not to spread the cells. The penis may also become infected with yeast. In one study, semen of the spouses of some women with recurrent yeast infections was found to contain yeast organisms thought to infect the seminal vesicles. Yeast was also found to colonize the mouths of husbands of some women with recurrent yeast vaginitis, suggesting that oral-genital contact might be a source of reinfection in such women. Treating the husbands systemically for yeast in these cases drastically reduced the incidence of vaginal infections in the wives.[7] To determine the presence of seminal yeast in the husband, a semen sample is required; prostatic fluid obtained by massaging the prostate gland through the rectal wall will not contain yeast from the seminal vesicles.[8] The only morally acceptable method of such semen collection is through the use of a perforated, non-spermicidal condom. This allows some semen to be deposited in the vagina and some to be retained for analysis.

Recurrent yeast infections are a prime symptom of candidiasis, or yeast overgrowth, which is believed by some doctors to affect many bodily functions. This newly discovered disease is discussed in Chapter 13 of this book. Dr. Trowbridge

* *See "Further Reading"*

includes a directory of "yeast-aware" doctors in his book; his directory would be an excellent way to locate a new physician if yeast infections continue to occur with traditional treatment.[9]

Bacterial Infections

Bacterial vaginosis is less common than yeast infection. It is characterized by a "foul or fishy-smelling, gray or yellowish vaginal discharge. Some women also suffer itching, low back pain, pain on urination, cramps, or irritation during intercourse."[10] IUDs and diaphragms may contribute to these infections, again illustrating the value of natural family planning in this regard.[11]

What can you do to prevent or get rid of a bacterial vaginal infection?

First of all, double-check your hygiene practices. The same irritating substances mentioned relative to yeast infections (feminine hygiene sprays, deodorant tampons, scented toilet paper, and so forth) should also be avoided in order to prevent bacterial infections. Menstrual pads are far preferable to tampons when bacterial infections are a problem. Wiping from front to back is a usual recommendation for preventing bacterial contamination from the feces. Since the cervical mucus helps protect against infection, the woman who is prone to bacterial infection should be especially careful during menstruation and during the "dry" times of the month.

Hygiene also applies to your love-making practices. The practice of male-to-female oral-genital contact as part of foreplay can transmit bacterial infections even if the husband is not aware of having them. One woman reported to the Couple to Couple League that she was troubled by recurrent bacterial vaginal infections until she and her husband completely stopped such oral-genital contact. Temporary cessation wasn't sufficient since apparently he was the unknowing host; she got rid of the infection but he apparently kept reinfecting her. Note also that the cold sore virus (Herpes I or herpes simplex) can also be transmitted in this way with roughly the same dangers as the Herpes II virus.

You might also consider nutritional aids, particularly **vitamin A**, if scant mucus is a problem (see Chapter 6, "Cycle Irregularities and Female Infertility," especially those subtopics which include scant mucus as a symptom). For postmenopausal women who experience vaginal irritation due to dryness, **vitamins A** and **E**, **zinc** and **selenium** may be helpful. Dr. Stuart Berger recommends 600 I.U. of vitamin E and 150 mcg of selenium daily for postmenopausal women.[12]

If you already have a vaginal bacterial infection, douching each evening for one week with a three percent solution of hydrogen peroxide diluted 1:4 with warm water may help to control a minor outbreak.[13] As with yeast infections, abstinence is advisable when bacterial infections are present. If antibiotic treatment is necessary, be aware of the possibility of yeast infection (see foregoing discussion, "Yeast Infections"). Husbands of women who are troubled by frequent bacterial infections of the vagina should be examined also and treated if infection of the penis or prostate is present (see "Prostatitis" in Chapter 12).[14]

Accurate diagnosis is essential for vaginal infections that do not quickly respond to home remedies. For those with reason to believe that their infection could be sexually transmitted, immediate medical diagnosis and treatment of both spouses by a careful, systematic physician is a must.

9

Pregnancy

The most fearful complication of pregnancy is eclampsia—convulsions that may occur in late pregnancy and which can be fatal to mother and child. Fortunately, eclampsia does not occur without warning, and that warning is the disease called toxemia (metabolic toxemia of late pregnancy, or preeclampsia, as it is also called). Toxemia can be recognized by high blood pressure and protein in the urine. For this reason prenatal care includes careful monitoring of both, especially during the last trimester. When early signs of toxemia occur, the woman is frequently advised to rest in order to help keep her blood pressure down, and to limit salt in order to reduce the edema (swelling) that precedes and accompanies toxemia. When the signs indicate serious toxemia, labor is frequently induced to prevent the dangerous eclampsia. While induction of labor is certainly preferable to possible life-threatening convulsions, such intervention has its own risks to mother and child. Avoiding the edema, toxemia and induction of labor is by far the best solution; yet toxemia is distressingly common even among women who are doing their best to have a healthy pregnancy, including taking their prescription prenatal vitamins.

What can you do to have a healthy pregnancy?
More specifically, what can you do to avoid recognized

problems for both yourself and your baby? I think the evidence is strong that there is a connection between good nutrition and avoiding such problems, so let's take a look at the evidence. Then you will be able to prepare yourself accordingly.

Texas physician John Ellis spent years studying the relationship between vitamin B_6 deficiency and various disorders including pregnancy edema, toxemia and eclampsia. Any woman who is interested in preventing these disorders would be well advised to read "B_6 During Pregnancy" in Dr. Ellis' book, *Vitamin B_6:The Doctor's Report.** The following excerpts from this book summarize the results of his clinical experience:

Numerous signs and symptoms appear during pregnancy that are responsive to B_6. These include painful neuropathies in the fingers and hands, swelling (edema) in the hands and feet, leg cramps, hand and arms "that go to sleep," and, most of all, B_6 is a factor in the prevention and treatment of toxemia of pregnancy and the convulsions of eclampsia...

Edema of pregnancy, long discussed in both medical and lay circles, has become so common that many doctors have come to accept it as being normal during pregnancy, and patients have grown resigned to suffering through it. *It is not normal at all. It is not normal at any time.* The patient feels bad. There is nothing healthy about being swollen with fluids.

Based on my investigations with 225 pregnant women on B_6 therapy, in most cases vitamin B_6 will completely relieve and prevent edema of pregnancy as it has been known to the scientific community. This is a large statement, but it has been proved over and over. Because of the skepticism that some readers may entertain, it would be wise to repeat that in these 225 cases *no diuretics were given to any patient, and there was no restriction on either salt or fluids.*[1]

Doctor Ellis presented a series of conclusions based on his research, including emphasis that salt restriction is not necessary when vitamin B_6 is adequate, and that the babies born to mothers who have taken large doses of B_6 do not show

* See "Further Reading"

increased need for this vitamin.[2] He also notes the role of magnesium, which works synergistically with vitamin B_6:

> ... All pregnant women should have at least 50 milligrams of B_6 [daily] as a supplement throughout their pregnancies, and many of them will require considerably more than that [he recommends up to 450 mg]. *All* pregnant women should also receive at least 500 milligrams of magnesium daily, and with the appearance of the signs of toxemia the magnesium should be increased to 1,000 milligrams daily.[3]

The following anecdote, contributed by a young medical student, may help illustrate the beneficial effects of proper nutrition during pregnancy:

> My wife and I were expecting our third child. Both of our older children had been born at home, and our plans were to deliver this child at home as well. However, a potentially serious problem presented an obstacle to a safe delivery at home. Despite care in maintaining good nutrition, in each of the other two pregnancies my wife had retained water and experienced nausea far beyond the normal length of "morning sickness." In addition, she had other related problems, such as tingling and numbness in her fingers and hands, joint aches and pains, elevated blood pressure, and a general feeling of not being well. These symptoms had occurred earlier in the second pregnancy than the first, and now, in the third, were occurring earlier still; she was only in the fourth month of pregnancy and had already gained 35 pounds. We both felt strongly that she had been only slightly better than a marginal candidate for home delivery with the last baby, and that if she wasn't in substantially better health with this pregnancy (largely because 6-1/2 years had passed, and she was now 30 years old with a family history of diabetes), it would not be safe to have this baby at home. However, we were even less enthusiastic about a hospital birth.
>
> As we were in the middle of this quandary, I had the opportunity to discuss the subject with the author, with whom I taught a class weekly. She shared with me information on the importance of good multi-vitamin supplements, and recommended an excellent non-prescription prenatal multi-vitamin, Magna Natal by Radiance.* [The full dose of this supplement (six tablets/day) contains 75 mg/

* See "Resources"

mcg of most B vitamins, 100 mg of B_6, 450 mg of magnesium, and other vitamins and minerals in amounts similar to those in Table 5, Chapter 3.]

As soon as my wife began taking these vitamins (and I mean within one day), she began shedding excess water, and experienced a visible improvement of the edema in her hands and feet. She lost nearly six pounds in the first week, and continued to improve until we could see the veins on the tops of her feet. Her blood pressure remained normal, there was no numbness, and she only occasionally felt nauseous. The improvement was so pronounced that we no longer felt reservations about continuing with plans for a home birth.

The effectiveness of this improvement in nutrition was demonstrated very pointedly some weeks later, when we ran out of the vitamin supplement, and found that the health food store where we had purchased them was also out of stock. In the week that my wife was not taking this supplement, she quickly became fatigued, nauseous, and edematous [swollen with fluid]. As soon as we had obtained a new supply and she had begun to take them regularly again, the problems disappeared.

My wife enjoyed excellent health throughout the remainder of the pregnancy, and delivered a bright, healthy baby boy at home.

I want to emphasize also that the needs for calories, protein, micronutrients and fluids all increase during pregnancy. Weight gain on nutritious food is central; I consider a thirty pound gain the bare minimum for a healthy pregnancy, and thin women often need to gain considerably more. *Failure to take in adequate calories and/or adequate protein is a leading cause of premature and low birth weight babies.* About 75 or 80 grams of protein should be consumed daily once the appetite allows, at least by the second trimester. This much protein is easy to eat if you have two four-ounce servings of meat per day (20 g each) and a quart of milk (30 g). Your other foods will easily make up the difference. Table 7, "Minimum Daily Food Goals for Pregnant and Nursing Women," is designed to help you meet your daily needs for protein and calories. The Nutrition Almanac* also has a section on the protein content of various foods.

* see "Further Reading"

94

The late nutritionist Adelle Davis, author of a series of popular books on diet and supplements, strongly believed that even the minor complaints of pregnancy—nausea, headache, fatigue, varicose veins, "mask" of pregnancy—are abnormalities that can be prevented or reversed with proper diet and supplements. I personally have found her book, *Let's Have Healthy Children,** to be indispensible during all of my pregnancies. Using the index, you can locate almost any disorder or annoyance of pregnancy and find several nutritional suggestions for overcoming it.

I have had excellent results with supplements similar to the higher doses listed in Table 5 (Chapter 3). I've had absolutely no puffiness of the hands or feet, except for one week of my fourth pregnancy when I discontinued all supplements just to observe the effect. I've been able to overcome disabling migraine headaches, which developed during my third and fourth pregnancies, by strictly avoiding sugar and caffeine and increasing folic acid to 3,000 or more mcg daily. I've nursed a toddler throughout my second, fourth and fifth pregnancies and certainly attribute my good health during this additional nutritional stress to careful supplementation and plenty of calories and protein. I have simply informed my prenatal physicians of my choice to use my own supplements instead of prescription prenatal vitamins, which I consider unbalanced and inadequate. For example, the typical prescription prenatal vitamin contains 3 to 10 mg of vitamin B_6 (the RDA is only 3 mg) and sometimes very little magnesium. (The reason for the medical prescription: they contain 1,000 mcg of folic acid which exceeds the statutory limits for nonprescription vitamins.)

* See "Further Reading"

Table 7
Minimum Daily Food Goals
for
Pregnant and Nursing Women

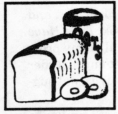

WHOLE GRAINS

4 servings daily (1 serving = 2 slices bread or 1/2 cup cooked cereal)

- Whole grain bread
- Oatmeal
- Whole grain breakfast cereal
- Whole grain pasta
- Whole grain pancakes
- Rice
- Millet
- Tortillas
- Bagels

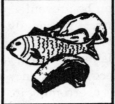

COMPLETE PROTEIN

2 servings daily (1 serving = 4 oz. meat)

- Poultry
- Fish (preferably twice weekly)
- Beef, including liver and heart
- Pork
- Lamb
- Grain + Legume (peas, beans, peanut butter, nuts, lentils)
- Dairy + Grain
- Dairy + Legume

☐ ☐ ☐ ☐   ☐ ☐

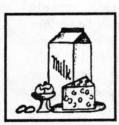

DAIRY\ EGGS

4 servings daily (1 serving = 8 oz. milk, 2 oz. cheese, 1 egg)

- Milk
- Yogurt
- Cheese
- Ice cream
- Kefir
- Eggs

YELLOW FRUITS AND VEGETABLES

5 servings *WEEKLY* (1 serving = 1/2 cup cooked or 1 cup raw)

- Carrots
- Squash
- Sweet Potatoes
- Pumpkin
- Cantaloupe
- Apricots
- Peaches

☐ ☐ ☐ ☐   ☐ ☐ ☐ ☐ ☐

Table 7, cont'd.

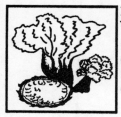

LEAFY GREEN VEGETABLES

2 servings daily
(1 serving =
1/2 cup cooked
or 1 cup raw)

- Lettuce (leaf, Romaine, bibb, iceberg)
- Spinach
- Escarole
- Endive
- Beet greens
- Alfalfa sprouts
- Cole crops (cabbage, broccoli, Brussels sprouts, cauliflower, kohlrabi)
- Asparagus
- Chard
- Kale

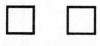

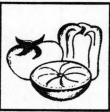

VITAMIN C SOURCE

1 serving daily
(1 serving =
1 medium fruit
or 1/2 cup berries)

- Citrus fruits (oranges, grapefruits, tangerines)
- Tomatoes
- Melons
- Berries
- Peppers
- Potatoes

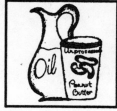

UNSATURATED OILS

1 serving daily
(1 serving =
1 - 2 tablespoons)

Polyunsaturated
- Safflower oil
- Sunflower oil
- Soy oil
- Corn oil

Monounsaturated
- Peanut oil
- Unprocessed peanut butter
- Olive oil
- Avocado oil

Both
- Sesame oil
- Canola oil

(Weekly intake should be approximately 50% polyunsaturated, 50% monounsaturated.)

NOTES

- Each type of food should be counted only once per day.
- This table may be photocopied, covered with adhesive-backed clear plastic and taped to your refrigerator. Check off the boxes daily with an erasable marker.
- Remember, your need for good food continues even if your appetite stops!

10

Repeated Miscarriage and Birth Defects

If you have had personal experience with either of these subjects, let me first say that I am sorry for the sadness it has brought you. I hope that you find courage in the face of this disappointment and heartache. Let me emphasize also that the purpose of this section is not to stir up "what if's" or "if only's." Very seldom can even experts know the underlying cause of a particular miscarriage or a particular birth defect, and even the most optimistic agree that not all prenatal loss or developmental errors will ever be prevented.

Nevertheless, is there anything you can do that might reduce the possibility of miscarriage and birth defects?

Once again, I think there's good evidence that optimal nutrition may be helpful. Promising new data indicate that certain micronutrients may play particularly critical roles in reducing the incidence of these two problems.

It appears that the ideal time to do our best to prevent miscarriage and birth defects is the three months prior to and immediately following conception. Early miscarriage may actually result from inadequate hormonal status preceding ovulation, and serious birth defects originate within the first eight weeks of pregnancy when organs are being formed. Ideally, the three months before conception should include attention to diet, supplements and body weight; it should also include the elimination of unhealthy practices such as smoking, drinking, and excessive caffeine and sugar consumption. As we will see, these pre-conception preparations are as important to the potential father as to the mother, and those of us in our family-forming years should make it a point to cultivate good diet and life-style habits, not only for our own sake but also for the sake of future children.

Miscarriage

Repeated early miscarriage is one manifestation of inadequate corpus luteal function.[1] Abnormal FSH or LH before ovulation apparently causes ovulation of an immature egg and/or the subsequent formation of a corpus luteum which releases insufficient progesterone for an insufficient number of days.[2] In such a situation pregnancy may be difficult to achieve; but even if it does occur, the newly conceived life may not be capable of normal development, or the corpus luteum may not produce enough of the progesterone necessary to sustain the pregnancy. The PMS nutritional strategy described in Chapter 5, "Premenstrual Syndrome," particularly "The PMS Diet" and "PMS Supplements," is specifically designed to improve luteal function and luteal levels of progesterone. In Chapter 6, "Cycle Irregularities and Female Infertility," the topic "Luteal Phase Inadequacy" explains the relationship between luteal function, fertility, and certain nutrients. This information is also pertinent to those who have experienced unexplained early miscarriage, especially if fetal development did not occur.

Joy DeFelice has found that eliminating night lighting from the woman's bedroom has improved short luteal phase manifestations and may prevent early miscarriage in many cases.[3] I believe that other factors which contribute to the inability to conceive such as being overweight or underweight or consuming excessive caffeine should also be remedied if possible by the woman whose infertility takes the form of miscarriage (see these topics in Chapter 6). It goes without saying that alcohol, nicotine and all but essential medications should be avoided, preferably by all those seeking pregnancy, but even more so by those parents, father and mother, who have experienced repeated miscarriages.

Adelle Davis in her book *Let's Have Healthy Children** calls special attention to the role of **vitamin E** and **folic acid** in preventing miscarriage:

A lack of vitamin E, essential to cell division, appears to be one of the most damaging [deficiencies]. In one study, 81 women who had suffered 227 previous miscarriages gave birth to 61 healthy babies after they had been given small amounts of vitamin E daily before the next conceptions. Among its important functions, vitamin E prevents the inactivation of **vitamin A**, which is necessary to maintain a healthy uterine lining to receive the newly fertilized egg....

Studies have shown that more than half the women who have miscarried or have had spotting during pregnancy show signs of folic acid deficiency... A deficiency of folic acid too mild to induce an abortion [miscarriage] can still cause the placenta to become detached from the uterine wall, a condition known as *abruptio placentae,* which is a common cause of premature births.[4]

Other **B vitamins**, **vitamin C**, the **bioflavinoids** (found in the white rind and segments of citrus fruits or available as supplements), **iodine, zinc** and adequate **protein** have also been related to the prevention of miscarriage in humans or experimental animals.[5] **Selenium** works synergistically with vitamin E and should also be considered. *Conversely, iron supplements destroy vitamin E and should not be taken in excessive amounts nor at the same time of day as vitamin E.* New Mexico physician Jack C. Redman has reported that 200 milligrams of bioflavinoids taken three times daily has prevented further miscarriages even in women who have experienced several. The bioflavinoids, which work together with vitamin C, apparently strengthen fragile capillary walls.[6]

* See "Further Reading"

Birth Defects

A very promising body of research points to the role of **folic acid** in preventing spina bifida and other common birth defects that are collectively referred to as "neural tube defects." Anencephaly, or failure of the brain to develop, is an even more severe neural tube defect than is spina bifida, and it is a major cause of stillbirth. In one large study, women who had previously had children born with one of these developmental errors received multi-vitamin supplements emphasizing folic acid (360 mcg/day) for at least four weeks prior to conception and for at least six weeks afterward. Only 0.6% of these mothers had another child with a neural tube defect, while 5% of a large group of unsupplemented mothers who had previously had a child with this defect had a second baby with a similar birth defect.[7] Similar studies in Great Britain have confirmed the role of folic acid (360-4,000 mcg/day) in significantly reducing recurrences of neural tube defects.[8] Related research has shown that improved diet alone can prevent recurrences of neural tube defects, though not necessarily to the same extent that was achieved in the studies using supplementation of folic acid.[9]

Since the large majority of cases of spina bifida, anencephaly and related disorders occur in mothers who have not previously borne a child with such a defect, research of neural tube defects involving general populations is of high interest. In one late eighties population-based study in the United States, mothers who had normal babies were significantly more likely to report taking multi-vitamin supplements during the three months before and the three months after conception than were mothers of children with neural tube defects.[10]

In a very large, carefully designed study of middle-class women in the Boston area, researchers found that babies of women who supplemented folic acid (100-1,000 mcg) in the first six weeks after conception had an incidence of neural tube defects of only 0.9 per thousand, while babies of mothers who did not supplement folic acid during the same six weeks had an incidence of neural tube defects of 3.5 per thousand—four times higher than the supplemented group.[11] This excellent study pinpointed the critical time period for preventing these types of birth defects with folic acid—the first six weeks after conception, which is when the involved neural structures are formed.

Promising preliminary data also show that large supplements of folic acid (10,000 mcg/day) before conception may reduce the risk of cleft lip in children of mothers who have had other children with this developmental problem.[12]

Deficiencies of **vitamins A, E, B₂, pantothenic acid, zinc** and **manganese** have all been linked to various types of developmental defects in animals, and in humans the incidence of congenital heart defects has increased at the same time that the American diet has become more deficient in vitamin E.[13] However, excessive vitamin A intake can *cause* birth defects; Dr. Marshall Mandell considers more than 100,000 I.U. per day dangerous,[14] but nutritionist Patricia Hausman reports a birth defect in a baby which may have been related to the mother's use of only 25,000 I.U. per day throughout the first three months of pregnancy and 50,000 I.U. thereafter.[15] Since vitamin A increases the need for vitamin E, I think this incident points out the need for balance of supplements.

It is my belief that the increased incidence of birth defects which is seen in the children of older mothers relates at least in part to increased nutritional needs as women grow older. I have seen this increased need personally. During my fourth pregnancy at age thirty-five, I developed folic acid deficiency anemia while taking one and one-half times the RDA for pregnant women for this vitamin; yet the same amount had been completely adequate during previous pregnancies. (Taking five times the RDA restored normal hematocrit values in four weeks during my seventh month of pregnancy.) I believe that all of us must conscientiously improve our nutrition year by year as we age if we expect to have the same sense of well-being and good health that we had five or ten or twenty years ago. This point is especially important, I think, for those of us who hope to have children in our late thirties or early forties, especially if we have had multiple pregnancies.

The Father's Role

The role of the father in miscarriage and birth defects is a factor which is infrequently considered. A long list of environmental toxins and drugs can cause sperm mutation—"heavy metals, pesticides, solvents, food additives and contaminants, alkylating agents, antibiotics and synthetic steroids."[16]

If mutated sperm fertilize an ovum, the most likely outcome is spontaneous abortion [miscarriage] insofar as all of the cells in the resulting embryo will have chromosomal anomalies. Other less likely outcomes include the occurrence of stillbirths, birth defects, and childhood diseases.[17]

Is there anything a man can do to avoid the sort of damage to his own fertility that may have these unhappy effects?

(Please note that the more general subject of male fertility and infertility is treated in Chapter 12.) Some things are a matter of common sense; in other matters, the evidence is suggestive.

Obviously, exposure to at least some of these toxins can be controlled. Furthermore, optimal nutrition with emphasis on whole foods and vitamin supplements, especially **vitamins A, C**, and **E** and the mineral **selenium**, can greatly assist the cells in eliminating harmful toxic byproducts. In laboratory animals, caffeine and alcohol cause pre- and post-implantation losses (miscarriages) in litters fathered by males treated with these chemicals.[18] Whether or not these substances affect early human pregnancy when used by the father before conception, this example illustrates that we certainly have the ability to control at least some factors that may adversely affect the ability to bear young. I believe that in any type of infertility, including repeated miscarriage, both parents should strive for the best nutrition possible, as outlined in Part I. They also need to keep in mind that it takes perhaps two months for improved nutrition practices to affect complete sperm development (see Chapter 12, "The Male Connection"). Once conception has occurred, the father's physical contribution to his child is complete, but his continued emphasis on good nutrition will not only enhance his own health; it is also the best encouragement to excellent nutrition that he can offer to his expectant wife.

11

The Premenopause

The permanent cessation of menses is termed the menopause; the transitional period of perhaps two years or twenty cycles before the final menses is called the premenopause. During the premenopause, the hormonal output from the ovaries gradually diminishes, though even after menopause both the ovaries and the adrenal glands continue to secrete reproductive hormones.

If you are a woman approaching the premenopausal years—from age forty to forty-nine or so—how should you prepare yourself nutritionally for this time of very high micronutrient needs?

Cycle irregularity of various types is probably inevitable for a while, but the nutritional strategies for irregular cycles should be implemented vigorously to limit the duration of this time (see Chapter 6, "Cycle Irregularities and Female Infertility"). You should especially prepare to avoid the three most distressing problems that may occur in the premenopause: very heavy, prolonged menses, hot flashes, and depression or other psychological symptoms. Heavy bleeding is covered separately (see Chapter 7), but the principles apply to the premenopausal woman as well, assuming, of course, that underlying pathology has been ruled out.

Vitamin E and **selenium** are commonly recommended for the annoying but harmless hot flashes that may occur during this time. Dr. Stuart Berger recommends 600 I.U. of vitamin E and 150 mcg of selenium daily for menopausal women.[1] Along with **vitamin A** and **zinc**, these may also help to alleviate vaginal dryness which often begins at this time of life.

The psychological symptoms which sometimes occur in the premenopausal time are rather similar to those reported by women with PMS. In fact, the PMS researchers Drs. Guy Abraham and Joel Hargrove suggest that "perimenopausal symptoms are just a continuation of PMT [PMS] symptoms and that therapy aimed at relieving PMT symptoms may be the best preventive measure against perimenopausal problems."[2] Dr. Hal Danzer recommends Dr. Abraham's nutritional strategy for premenopausal women over thirty-five.[3] Dr. Hargrove reports that women who implement Abraham's diet and supplement program need less estrogen replacement than others.[4] (See Chapter 6, especially "The PMS Diet" and "PMS Supplements.") This is a significant issue for any woman considering estrogen replacement therapy; smaller amounts of estrogen reduce the risk of cancer associated with estrogen treatment. Since body fat is the main source of estrogen after menopause,[5] the common tendency for slim women to gain a modest amount of weight around the time of menopause may actually be beneficial.

While **calcium** and **vitamin D** are important in preventing osteoporosis in later years, calcium must always be balanced with **magnesium**, which in turn enables the body to use calcium. Any additional calcium should be increased gradually, at a rate of 250 mg every four months or so, because large amounts of calcium may cause irritability and nervousness.[6] I would suggest that 250 mg of calcium be subtracted from the supplemental intake for each cup of milk in the diet and that the ratio of *total* calcium (dairy plus supplements) to *supplemental* magnesium equal 1:1.

Of particular concern to women in the premenopause and afterward is avoiding unnecessary hysterectomy. The overuse of this surgery has frequently been criticized. The late Dr.

Robert Mendelsohn estimated that only one of every five hysterectomies is medically justified.[7] Aside from the general risks that any major surgery entails, removal of the uterus can adversely affect a woman's sexual responsiveness, as in some women the cervix is sexually sensitive to penile pressure during intercourse.[8] If the ovaries, which produce significant amounts of androgens ("male" hormones), are also removed, sexual desire may drop since these hormones are responsible for the sexual appetite in both men and women.[9] Heavy bleeding is all too often treated with hysterectomy during the premenopause; yet as Chapter 7 points out, this problem can often be solved by careful nutrition. Larrian Gillespie, M.D., a woman urologist, makes a strong case that hysterectomy is frequently recommended by gynecologists when it is the bladder that actually requires treatment.[10] She recommends that women thoroughly investigate this possibility with a qualified urologist before undergoing hysterectomy. I refer to her book, *You Don't Have to Live With Cystitis!** reluctantly— the tone, examples and illustrations frequently offend modesty and morality. However, it contains the best information I have seen on this topic, as well as excellent information on urinary tract infections.

* *See "Further Reading"*

12

The Male Connection

While everyone recognizes the role of the man in conceiving children, when it comes to infertility, the primary emphasis has been on the role of the woman. To a certain extent, that may be justified by the fact that the female reproductive system is more complicated and must contribute not only to conception but also to implantation and carrying the baby. However, in recent years, more emphasis has been given to the role of the husband in cases of infertility, and I believe that the evidence indicates that there is a definite connection between nutrition and male fertility. Certain nutrition and health practices may also help to alleviate a bothersome condition called prostatitis.

Male Infertility

"Quality and quantity"—this expression is often used by reproductive physiologists to summarize the essentials of male fertility. It refers, of course, to the male reproductive cells, the sperm.

The quality of the sperm refers to their ability to move forward, to contribute to digesting away the tissue surrounding the ovum, and to engage in actual fertilization. Quality can be judged by microscopically observing the shape (morphology) of the sperm as well as their movements (motility). The majority should have a normal head and a long, single tail; abnormalities such as double heads or short, twisted tails should be relatively few in number. Most sperm should be capable of forward movement by the whipping motion of the tail, and clumping of the sperm, or spermagglutination, should not occur in more than a fourth of the sperm cells.

The quantity of sperm necessary for normal fertility is one of those numbers that physiology professors love to use to awe their students. Each of the three or four milliliters of ejaculated semen typically contains from sixty to one hundred twenty *million* sperm. When the sperm count drops to "only" twenty million per milliliter, the man is usually infertile.[1] These numbers seem to be necessary to overcome the somewhat acidic environment of the vagina, to compensate for loss as sperm migrate throughout the female reproductive tract, and to provide for adequate numbers if ovulation occurs two or three days after intercourse. Thousands of sperm must arrive in the vicinity of the ovum to chemically digest its covering before the nucleus of a single sperm can fuse to the nucleus of the ovum, an event that begins the life of a new individual.

The sheer amount of cellular synthesis of sperm occurring within the seminiferous tubules of the testes suggests the high nutrient needs of these glands. The active motion required of sperm also implies a high requirement of these cells for the micronutrients that contribute to liberating cellular energy. And since sperm production depends on hormonal stimulation by FSH, LH and testosterone, the nutrients that are involved in hormone synthesis are necessarily involved in male fertility.

What can a man do to promote his own fertility, and what can he do if he is subfertile?

The evidence suggests that optimal nutrition assists normal fertility and that supplements can sometimes remedy certain types of infertility.

In one of the most dramatic studies ever published on the effect of nutrition on reproductive function, twenty-seven men with infertility apparently due to spermagglutination were divided into two groups. Twenty received supplemental **vitamin C** (1,000 mg/day) plus calcium, magnesium and manganese (all found in the Shaklee Vita-C tablets used in this research).

Following the 60-day regimen, all subjects were re-examined for evidence of change. The wives of each of the twenty men who received supplemental ascorbic acid [vitamin C] had become pregnant during the study period. In contrast, no wife of any subject in the group which did not receive supplemental doses had become pregnant during this time period.[2]

This program of supplementation significantly improved sperm quantity, morphology and motility, and reduced spermagglutination.[3] A subsequent study used pure vitamin C (200 or 1,000 mg/day) and confirmed the beneficial effect of this nutrient on the same measures of fertility in men with spermagglutination.[4] In only one week, sperm counts for those receiving 1,000 mg/day of vitamin C rose an average of 140%![5] "The results of this study . . . provide direct evidence of the importance of AA [ascorbic acid; vitamin C] in maintaining physiological integrity of the testis, epididymus, and accessory glands."[6] Testosterone production also depends on the presence of vitamin C.[7]

Zinc is another nutrient which is absolutely essential for synthesis of testosterone by the testes. In men with kidney failure (who lose zinc excessively in the urine) but maintained by kidney machine, 50 mg of zinc per day given under double-blind conditions improved potency, sexual desire and frequency of intercourse.[8] "Mild" cases of zinc deficiency have caused low sperm counts in men,[9] and supplemental zinc has increased testosterone levels and sperm counts in infertile men.[10] The highest concentrations of zinc in the body are found in the sperm cells and in the prostate gland; this gland's health contributes importantly to male reproductive capability.

Vitamin A, which aids the lining membranes throughout the body, similarly benefits the lining cells of the testes' seminiferous tubules—and these cells are the developing sperm!

Males are more sensitive, in general, than are females, to the lack of vitamin A . . . In man, blood and kidney levels of vitamin A are higher in males and men are more prone to develop night blindness. In experimentally induced deficiency of vitamin A, varying degrees of atrophy [shrinkage] of the epididymus, seminal vesicle and prostate gland have been reported. In severe deficiency there is degeneration of the seminiferous tubules, a reduction of semen volume and of sperm count and motility, and an increased proportion of abnormal spermatic forms.[11]

A lack of the B vitamins can cause a reduction of pituitary function, which is necessary to produce the LH and FSH which stimulate sperm production and testosterone secretion. In animals at least, deficiencies of the **B vitamins (B_1, B_2, B_6, B_{12}), pantothenic acid, biotin** and **folic acid** have all been shown to damage the testes or other reproductive organs.[12]

Several other nutrients may also affect male fertility. Male animals have a higher need than females for essential fatty acids, including **linoleic acid** and arachidonic acid.[13] The former is abundant in **safflower oil**, and perhaps one to two tablespoons per day of this oil should be eaten as part of the salad dressing. Arachidonic acid is usually excessive in American diets since it is found in red meats; in reality it should be limited. At least in rats, selenium deficiency causes immobile sperm with fragile tails that break off.[14]

Doctor Stuart Berger emphasizes the role of **vitamins B_{12}, C** and **E**, and the minerals **zinc** and **selenium** in male reproductive function.[15] He recommends that men take 600 I.U. of vitamin E, 100 mg of zinc, and 150 mcg of selenium daily.[16] With reference to the latter mineral,

...almost half of your body's supply of selenium is located in your testicles and the seminal ducts next to your prostate gland. Your sperm cells also include significant amounts of the mineral, so each time you ejaculate, you lose a quantity of selenium. That means you have to keep replacing it, to assure optimal sexual functioning.[17]

Keep in mind that selenium can be toxic; Dr. Berger recommends 300 mcg as a maximum dose.[18]

Prescription drugs, workplace toxins and alcohol can all lower male fertility or sperm counts.[19] Alcohol decreases levels of testosterone, ultimately contributing to lowered sperm production *which may be irreversible*.[20] The effects of caffeine on male fertility in the human have not been directly studied although the late eighties' finding that caffeine reduces female fertility will surely lead to investigations of this question in the nineties (see "Caffeine Consumption" in Chapter 6). There are data from animal studies suggesting that caffeine does affect testicular function, including a study in roosters in which caffeine caused lowered fertility progressing to complete cessation of testicular function.[21] Based on the latter study, these researchers hypothesize that caffeine consumption in men of 600 mg/day (about six cups of coffee daily) could adversely affect male fertility, especially in those who already have a low sperm count.[22] I strongly encourage men with infertility of any cause to sharply reduce or eliminate caffeine, alcohol, nicotine and all but essential medicines. Part I outlines the basics of good diet, and the supplements listed in Table 5 (Chapter 3) will "cover all the bases" of micronutrient needs for male fertility.

It is useful to realize that sperm require over two months to mature; therefore, improvement of male fertility through nutrition may not occur immediately (except possibly in the case of spermagglutination and vitamin C). And it should be emphasized that whenever infertility is a problem, *both* spouses should improve their nutrition and both should employ *all* the fertility techniques taught by the Couple to Couple League.* One can rarely know with absolute certainty which spouse's reproductive dysfunction underlies the infertility, and often it is both spouses'. Attempting to optimize

* See "Resources"

reproductive health through nutrition may also enable one spouse to compensate for the other's subfertility. For example, the wife's attempting to increase cervical mucus with vitamin A may help to overcome infertility due to low sperm count in the husband, and if excellent nutrition raises a man's sperm count to higher levels, it could aid the problem of partially blocked uterine tubes in the woman. For these reasons I refer the reader to Chapter 6, "Cycle Irregularities and Female Infertility."

What if the problem is low sexual desire or impotence?

Assuming psychological factors are not the root cause, nutrition could be of value. **Zinc** (50 mg/ day) given under double-blind conditions has specifically helped men with such dysfunction,[23] but I suspect that all of the above-mentioned nutrients that improve sperm counts and testosterone levels would also be helpful. And since the health of the prostate gland importantly affects the ability to maintain an erection, the following section should also be seriously considered.

Prostatitis

A large number of urologists' patients are men with acute or chronic prostatitis. Prostatitis refers to infection or inflammation of the prostate gland, which is a disorder completely different from the benign prostatic hypertrophy (enlargement) that commonly causes problems in men over age fifty. The symptoms of prostatitis include pain between the legs or in the rectal area; sometimes this pain occurs with intercourse. More severe infection causes pain in the urethra and frequency of urination.

The usual medical treatment for prostatitis is antibiotic therapy. However, the infective microorganisms are notoriously difficult to eradicate and long-term treatment is often necessary. Many urologists routinely advise increased frequency of intercourse to "flush out" the gland, which empties its secretions into the urethra during coitus. The problem that

116

this poses to the couple practicing periodic abstinence needs no elaboration, and masturbation is immoral. Fortunately, a number of natural strategies can immensely help the prostatitis-prone man to prevent the troublesome flare-ups.

What are the self-help steps available to the man who is attempting to overcome or prevent recurring bouts of prostatitis?

1. *Avoid foods that produce an irritating urine.* Spicy or acid foods can cause intense attacks of prostatitis within hours. Condiments such as mayonnaise, ketchup, mustard, relish and so forth should be avoided. Tomatoes, raw onions, wieners, pizza, tacos, soft drinks, tea, coffee and alcohol are other culprits. Sometimes food additives in processed items cause reactions that home-cooked equivalent dishes do not.

2. *Improve blood flow to the prostate gland.* Exercise— especially running, boxer shorts instead of jockey briefs, and hot baths all aid circulation to this gland. Conversely, cigarette smoking, prolonged sitting and constipation impede its blood flow. Avoid nasal sprays and other cold or allergy remedies which constrict nasal tissues—they do the same to prostate vessels, and infections thrive where blood flow is poor.[24]

3. *Avoid urine backflow* into the prostatic ducts. The bladder should be emptied regularly and not allowed to become overfull. "Shy bladder" is common among men with prostatitis, and relaxation, not straining, should be practiced when urine is voided.

4. *Nourish the prostate properly.* **Zinc** is highly concentrated in this gland, and 100 mg per day of supplemental zinc may be helpful.[25] **Vitamins E** and **B$_6$** are also specifically recommended for prostatitis.[26] **Selenium** is important to all of the male reproductive organs. A diet low in saturated fats and adequate in unsaturated oils such as safflower or soy contributes to overall prostate health and may possibly help prevent enlargement of the gland as aging continues.

Chronic prostatitis may be a symptom of the yeast overgrowth disorder, candidiasis. See Chapter 13, "Candidiasis," for further information on this subject.

13

Candidiasis

Premenstrual syndrome, vaginal infections, menstrual pain, cycle irregularity, female infertility and chronic prostatitis have all been linked to the newly recognized and still controversial disorder, candidiasis. This disease, also called yeast overgrowth, is the abnormal transformation and proliferation of the usually harmless fungus, *Candida albicans,* within the body. Yet another name for such yeast infestation is polysystemic chronic candidiasis, emphasizing its potential to affect virtually all systems of the body over a prolonged period of time.

The symptoms of yeast overgrowth are numerous and diverse, according to doctors who accept candidiasis as a real, treatable disease. In addition to the reproductive system problems listed above, they include:

• Extreme fatigue or lethargy (the feeling of being drained)
• Depression
• Inability to concentrate
• Headaches
• Skin problems (such as hives, athlete's foot...)
• Gastrointestional problems (especially constipation, abdominal pain, diarrhea, gas or bloating...)
• Muscular and nervous system symptoms (including aching or swelling in your muscles and joints, numbness, burning or tingling...)

- Respiratory symptoms
- Hyperactivity and recurrent ear problems...[1]

In women, repeated vaginal yeast infections are a major sign of this disorder. Its symptoms also overlap markedly with those of PMS, though candidiasis does not show the clear-cut cyclicity characteristic of PMS. Some physicians have found that anti-candida treatment is very beneficial for PMS.[2] The strong link to reproductive dysfunction in women makes this disorder well worth considering in any woman who feels unexplainably unwell over a prolonged period, or who is unable to overcome the reproductive abnormalities which have been associated with candidiasis.

Women are more prone to yeast overgrowth than are men or children, but chronic prostatitis is a significant clue to its presence in a man. Dr. John Trowbridge offers an instructive anecdote illustrating a typical case of a young man's candida-induced prostatitis which followed antibiotic treatment.[3]

The chief predisposing factors involved in yeast overgrowth are as follows:

1. A history of antibiotic treatment... Longterm treatment with antibiotics can destroy many of the bacteria normally present in the digestive tract or vagina, bacteria that tend to discourage yeast growth...

2. Use of oral contraceptives. In some women, the synthetic estrogen and progestogens in birth control pills cause changes in the vaginal mucous membrane which allow yeasts to multiply more rapidly, causing vaginitis...

3. Cortisone, prednisone, or other corticosteroids... Steroids suppress or weaken the immune response, paving the way for yeast overgrowth.

4. Dietary factors... A diet high in sugary, starchy foods can cause yeast to multiply more rapidly, as the yeast feeds on sugar...

5. Multiple pregnancies.[4]

What can you do if you think you are troubled by candidiasis?

First of all, you should seek medical assistance if you have reason to believe that your poor health may be caused by candidiasis. While it is still considered a speculative disease by the American Academy of Allergy and Immunology, a growing number of medical and osteopathic doctors do treat this illness. You may contact such a "yeast-aware" physician by consulting the state-by-state listing in *The Yeast Syndrome.**

Second, modify your diet. Just as diet is implicated in the cause of candidiasis, it is central to its control. The anti-candida diet works on the principles of cutting off the yeast's food supply (sugar and starches), reducing the intake of yeast-containing foods, and providing the body with excellent nutrition to bolster the immune system. Thus sugar, honey, sweet fruits, refined carbohydrates and sometimes even "healthy" carbohydrates such as whole grains are eliminated, at least for a while. Yeast-containing breads, condiments, fruit juices, processed meats, alcohol and mushrooms are eliminated, at least temporarily. Dr. Trowbridge calls this restrictive early diet "MEVY," for meat, eggs, vegetables and yogurt, the foods which are permissible or, in the case of yogurt, especially beneficial. He considers this diet almost as helpful as the anti-fungal drug, nystatin, in counteracting candidiasis.[5]

Third, consider food supplements. **Magnesium**, **vitamin B**$_6$, and fatty acids such as those found in **fish oils** and **flaxseed oil** are thought to prevent candidiasis or to promote healing of it. **Vitamin A** (but not its precursor, beta-carotene) may be useful for treating candidiasis.[6] Multi-vitamins and minerals in amounts roughly equivalent to those in Table 5 (Chapter 3) are also recommended by doctors who treat this disease.[7] Other nutritional supplements that are often recommended to combat yeast infestation are tablets of **acidophilus** ("friendly" bacteria), **aged garlic extract**, **aloe vera**, and **taheebo tea**.[8] All are available at better health food shops. Diet and supplements alone may control moderate cases of yeast, but severe overgrowth requires management with anti-candida drugs as well as strict dietary measures. In my opinion, generous intake of acidophilus tablets is the most

* *See "Further Reading"*

beneficial nonprescription therapy available, as the following anecdote illustrates.

An otherwise healthy thirty-five-year-old man related the following experience. After developing chronic prostatitis he had taken "ten different courses of antibiotics within two and a half years." The bouts were occurring more and more frequently, longer treatment with antibiotics was required, and finally, a course of antibiotics did no good at all. During this time he gradually realized that certain foods triggered these attacks—soda pop, alcohol, processed meats, condiments and most other processed foods. By strictly avoiding these he could control the prostatitis, but he felt he was "always on the razor's edge" if he ate the wrong food. He learned from Dr. William Crook's *The Yeast Connection* that chronic prostatitis is a possible symptom of candidiasis, and, in fact, he recalls, during his final few flare-ups his urologist could not culture bacteria from his prostatic fluid. He tried eating plain yogurt and noticed that it somewhat reduced the constant inflammation that troubled him. Reasoning that yogurt bacteria are largely killed off by the stomach's acid, he tried capsules of acidophilus, which are designed to release the friendly bacteria into the intestine, where they combat yeast. They helped immensely. He has not had a major recurrence nor used antibiotics for eighteen months, and he considers the low-level inflammation "virtually gone." Along with five capsules of acidophilus daily, he takes vitamins and minerals and eats only low-sugar, unprocessed foods, except for occasional treats. Testing has confirmed that he is highly allergic to yeast, but he believes that medical treatment is unnecessary at this time. He reports that he feels better now than before the prostatitis started, and jokes that he is "forced to eat only healthy food," though his sensitivity to many of his former "trigger" foods has decreased markedly. One can only speculate about how his problem would have progressed had he not on his own found "the yeast connection."

For a brief, clear discussion of yeast overgrowth, see "The Phantom Yeast: The Candida Connection" in Dr. Stuart

Berger's *What Your Doctor Didn't Learn in Medical School.**
For completely documented, exhaustive information on this
subject, refer to Dr. William Crook's *The Yeast Connection** or
to *The Yeast Syndrome,** by Dr. John Trowbridge and Morton
Walker.

* See "Further Reading"

14

Questions and Answers

• I have PMS, and my doctor has me on Optivite
three times a day. But when I feel good I forget
to take them, and when I feel bad, it's too late!
Any suggestions?

Yes, I do have one that works wonderfully. If you are
married, ask your husband to take sincere responsibility for
getting your vitamins out and reminding you to take them. If
you're single, ask your mother, sister or roommate to help you
in this way. This situation is very common among PMS
sufferers, and those who live with you will probably be glad to
help! For your part, respond maturely to their support.

If you live alone, place your vitamins where you will
remember to take them—for example, in the bathroom so you
can make them part of your after breakfast teeth-brushing
routine. Or have a trusted friend at work remind you—then
don't let her down. Incidentally, Procycle is very similar to
Optivite, but the entire day's dose is taken in the morning.

• We are postponing a pregnancy now using NFP.
But I've got mucus from the time my period ends

until I ovulate on day 25 or 30 or so. We would need to abstain a lot less if I didn't have such a long patch of mucus every month.

Improved nutrition can possibly help you, and either a shorter mucus patch or a shorter cycle length will make a difference. I would like to provide you with a checklist to help you identify possible causes of the long cycles and/or prolonged mucus. Then, you can refer to the appropriate subsections in Chapter 6 (or other chapters as noted) for specific nutritional aids. Keep in mind that more than one cause could apply to your situation. If so, do not "double up" on the suggested supplements. Just cover all the bases using Table 5 (Chapter 3) as a guide.

___ 1. Are you nursing a baby? Have you discontinued nursing within your last three cycles? The cycle characteristics you describe are normal for cycling, nursing mothers, but "classic" cycle patterns are equally normal if you are nursing only a little. You can encourage your reproductive hormones to complete the transition from breastfeeding subfertility to full fertility with excellent diet and supplements. Table 7 (Chapter 9), "Minimal Food Goals for Pregnant and Nursing Women," will be helpful if you are nursing a great deal; see Table 4 (Chapter 1), "Minimum Daily Food Goals" if you are nursing very little or have weaned. Supplements as in Table 5 (Chapter 3) should be considered, and be very sure that **vitamins A** and **E**, the **B vitamins** and **iodine** are well supplied. Magna Natal by Radiance Products* is excellent for both pregnant and nursing women.

___ 2. Have you recently discontinued birth control pills? If you have taken birth control pills recently, it's possible that their residual effects are still affecting you. It often takes up to four cycles for mucus patterns to become normal after discontinuing birth control pills, and I have talked to women who believe that various negative effects have persisted for years after they went off the Pill. (See "Discontinuing Birth

* *See "Resources"*

126

Control Pills" which will also direct you to the PMS nutritional plan in Chapter 5.)

___ 3. Are you in your mid-to-late forties? Premenopausal cycle changes could account for this pattern. See Chapter 11, "The Premenopause" for nutritional suggestions for this time of life. "The PMS Diet" and "PMS Supplements" (Chapter 5) may be particularly helpful in limiting the duration of cycle irregularity.

___ 4. Are you slender or underweight, even a little bit? Do you exercise vigorously? Have you dieted recently? (See "Underweight or Too Trim.")

___ 5. Are you obese or substantially overweight? (See "Overweight.")

___ 6. Do you drink more than one cup of coffee a day, or the equivalent in tea or caffeinated soda pop? Are you eating chocolate almost daily? (See "Caffeine Consumption.")

___ 7. Are your preovulatory basal temperatures around 97.4°F. or lower? You could have a slight tendency to low thyroid function—certainly not enough to cause a disease, but perhaps enough to explain your prolonged mucus and delayed ovulation. (See "Low Thyroid Function.")

___ 8. Is your luteal phase usually less than twelve days from the first day of temperature shift up to and including the last day before your period begins? (See "Luteal Phase Inadequacy," which will also direct you to the PMS nutritional plan in Chapter 5.)

___ 9. Could you be **vitamin A** deficient? Another sign of this is heavy or prolonged menses. If you do not eat many green or yellow vegetables and do not supplement vitamin A, consider this a possibility. (See "Other Causes of Poor Mucus Patterns, Cycle Irregularities or Infertility.")

___ 10. Is there any light at all in your bedroom at night? Some women's mucus patterns improve when night lighting in their bedrooms is eliminated or controlled. (See "Sensitivity to Night Lighting.")

___ 11. None of the above applies. If so, I strongly recommend that you try the PMS diet and supplement plan as outlined in Chapter 5 under the headings "The PMS Diet" and "PMS Supplements." If you are slender but not really underweight, try gaining just two or three pounds. Make sure that you are getting sufficient **iodine** (150 mcg/day) and **vitamin E** (400-600 I.U./day). Finally, give the night lighting strategy a try. (See "Sensitivity to Night Lighting.")

If these suggestions will make a difference, they certainly will do so within three to six months.

• I quit nursing my baby eighteen months ago, but my breasts have still not completely dried up, and my luteal phase is still short.

Galactorrhea, or milk in the breasts of non-nursing women, is not uncommon among those who have been pregnant. It most often indicates excessive prolactin secretion, or it can be a symptom of hypothyroidism, or, more rarely, hyperthyroidism.[1] These topics are discussed in Chapter 6, "Cycle Irregularities and Female Infertility" under the headings "Luteal Phase Inadequacy," "Low Thyroid Function," and "Hyperthyroidism." An evaluation by an endocrinologist (a doctor who specializes in hormonal disorders) can and should be made to determine the cause of galactorrhea, but the temperature chart itself contributes to the diagnosis. Very low or very elevated waking temperatures suggest, respectively, low or elevated levels of thyroid hormone. A short luteal phase is strong evidence of high prolactin levels.

The nutritional suggestions for lowering prolactin are listed under "Elevated Levels of the Hormone Prolactin" in Chapter 5. **Vitamin E** is also beneficial to breast tissue, and conversely, caffeine irritates it. Red meat and sugar should be limited also.

I suspect that in this situation fairly high amounts of vitamin B_6 (300-600 mg/day) may be necessary to lower prolactin levels significantly, but **magnesium** in generous amounts (800-1,000 mg/day) may make less B_6 necessary. One or two tablespoons of unrefined, unheated **safflower oil** should be taken daily, and **evening primrose oil** may be useful also. Nutritional and medical counseling is essential under these circumstances, but vitamins and minerals are natural substances that will get at the underlying cause, and are far preferable to the synthetic drug bromocriptine (Parlodel) which specifically lowers prolactin. Refer your counselors to the research of E.N. McIntosh, who found that vitamin B_6 alone eliminated the galactorrhea and amenorrhea caused by prolactin excess.[2]

You may be surprised to learn that galactorrhea is frequently undetected by women who have this condition.[3] Careful expression of each breast, from edge to nipple, should be part of routine breast self-examination. Even a single drop of fluid should be reported to a doctor, unless you are pregnant or nursing has been discontinued recently.

• My breasts hurt so much sometimes that I can't even hug my husband. Other times they feel uncomfortably full, but I'm not nursing. Please don't tell me it's my coffee—I'll give up anything else!

It probably is caffeine, as you've no doubt suspected by the correlation between your coffee habit and your symptoms. Cutting out caffeine is the primary dietary change that will help you. **Vitamin E** (400-600 I.U./day) is also useful for painful, polycystic breast disease. And you may notice that sugar bingeing causes water retention in a day or two; that retained fluid further aggravates breast tenderness. Since this problem is a common PMS symptom, the PMS nutritional strategy is well worth considering. (See Rule 5, Chapter 1, and Chapter 5, "Premenstrual Syndrome.")

• I never had a bladder infection until I got married,

but now I've had several. The doctor actually calls it "honeymoon cystitis." How can this be prevented?

There are nutritional guidelines as well as some considerations for during and after sexual intercourse that will help prevent recurrences. Both are aimed at reducing irritation of the bladder and/or urethra.

In women, who are far more prone to bacterial bladder infections (cystitis) than are men, the urethral opening lies close to the clitoris, and it can be irritated by too vigorous stimulation, either manually or genitally. Oral stimulation should be completely avoided. Urinating shortly after intercourse is very important, as is emptying the bladder every two hours or so during the day. This flushes away bacteria and prevents overstretch of the bladder, which reduces its blood supply. Drinking plenty of pure water dilutes the urine and encourages emptying.[4]

The commonly recommended cranberry juice is the worst possible remedy for bladder infections! Yes, it somewhat inhibits bacteria, but cranberry "drink" is loaded with sugar, and any acid or spicy food can irritate the urinary tract, allowing bacteria to take over. Tomato, mustard, Mexican or Italian food, soft drinks, coffee, tea and alcohol are troublemakers for those with this problem. Dr. Larrian Gillespie, in *You Don't Have to Live With Cystitis!*, lists many foods, including quite a few fruits, that exacerbate cystitis.[5] Her recommendations for supplements are fairly similar to those in Table 5 (Chapter 3).[6] **Vitamin C** in particular may be beneficial in preventing this problem.

If a bladder infection makes urination excruciating, pour a large glass of warm water slowly over the vulva as you void. Those who have had such infections report that this is a tremendous help.

• Morning sickness has made me miserable for the entire first three months of my pregnancies. What can help next time?

Clearly the dramatic changes in several hormones during early pregnancy are related to morning sickness, but exactly why the stomach becomes so hypersensitive and irritated is not well understood. Morning sickness is not in the least psychological—it is usually caused by stomach irritation and possibly by stimulation of the brain center that causes vomiting. And it is certainly not a "healthy sign," as some doctors tell women. Yes, it does indicate hormonal change, but many women, myself included, have had several pregnancies without even an hour of this distressing, demoralizing condition.

Vitamin B$_6$ is well known as the anti-nausea vitamin, and **magnesium** enhances its effect. (I've seen recommendations of 30 to 100 mg/day of the former; 500 mg/day of magnesium would be a reasonable supplement.) While vitamins are helpful, supplements can further irritate the stomach unless taken on a full stomach during your "best" time of day. Ideally, these and other vitamins would be started before conception.

Ginger root, the same spice found in your kitchen cupboard, is wonderful for all kinds of nausea. Capsules of ground ginger root are available at health food shops and can be taken with meals or made into a tea.

Other tips include limiting fatty and spicy foods, keeping food in the stomach, and taking fluids between meals, not with them. Water can make nausea worse; herbal mint tea may be helpful. Toast and crackers seem to help some women.

• How can I handle migraine headaches without medication?

The answer is to prevent them, and diet and supplements are extremely valuable for doing so. First, look for "triggers" and eliminate them whenever possible. Bright lights, certain odors such as those from cleaning agents, fuel stations, new carpets, cigarette smoke and other sources, and foods that contain the amino acid tyramine—aged cheeses, wine, beer—are possible culprits for precipitating migraine. Other foods may also trigger migraines. Eliminate completely the caffeine sources (coffee, tea, chocolate, cola and some medicines), but do so gradually since sudden withdrawal may cause an attack.

Hypoglycemia is closely related to migraine, and avoiding blood sugar swings is extremely important. Eating protein or complex carbohydrate snacks, avoiding alcohol, and limiting simple sugars are all helpful. Even sweet fruits can trigger a migraine, and all sweets should be eaten cautiously and on a full stomach only.

The **B vitamins** are valuable in maintaining normal blood glucose levels. **Folic acid** (2,000-3,000 mcg/day) is particularly helpful when taken with general supplements as suggested in Table 5 (Chapter 3).

• What are the nutritional guidelines for preventing breast cancer?

Doctor Guy Abraham points out that the risk of breast cancer is five times higher in those who have the luteal phase hormonal profile typical of many women with PMS—high estrogen and low progesterone.[7] He believes that his nutritional strategy for PMS, which lowers estrogen and elevates progesterone, will prevent many cases of breast cancer (see Chapter 5, particularly "The PMS Diet"). His plan is really just a variation on the "high fiber-low fat" diet that others also recommend for preventing breast cancer.

Obesity is a risk factor for breast cancer, probably because fat cells change androgens ("male" hormones) into estrogens, and elevated estrogens are associated with this type of cancer. Long-term nursing of babies reduces the risk of breast cancer, possibly because of the suppression of estrogen during this time.

• As a mother of five who has nursed for a total of

eight years, I am very concerned about osteoporosis. Yet from what I read, calcium alone doesn't seem to be the answer.

You are correct; studies on the effects of calcium supplementation on the bone loss disorder, osteoporosis, have not been especially promising. Both **vitamin D** and **magnesium** are necessary for the body to use **calcium,** and it is well to remember that sugar increases loss of **magnesium**.

Doctor Guy Abraham, whose outstanding work has done much to increase our understanding of the role of magnesium, states the following:

In certain parts of Asia and Africa, where predominantly vegetarian diets contain as little as 300-500 mgm of calcium/day, but with as much as 1,000 mgm of magnesium/day, osteoporosis is no more common than in Europe and North America where consumption of dairy products contributes to more than 1,000 mgm of calcium/day, but with intake of magnesium ranging from 143 to 300 mgm/day. Vegetarian women have a lower incidence of osteoporosis than omnivorous women. Recent evidence suggests that osteoporotic patients have a deficiency of...[vitamin D_3]... Administration of...[vitamin D_3] to such patients results in increased calcium absorption and retention. A diet high in magnesium and low in calcium with a magnesium/calcium ratio of at least 2:1 would enhance the formation of...[vitamin D_3], and therefore, increases the adaptability to low calcium intake. Such an approach would seem more physiological in the prevention of osteoporosis than using massive doses of calcium which suppresses formation of...[vitamin D_3].[8]

• On your tape from the Couple to Couple League 1988 Convention, you mentioned in passing that you have carpal tunnel syndrome, but you control it with nutrition. Could you give more details?

Carpal tunnel syndrome refers to pain, weakness and

numbness of the hands, wrists and sometimes elbows and shoulders. It's been shown in double-blind studies to respond to **vitamin B$_6$** supplements alone.[9] I've found that **magnesium** and **vitamin C** also help, especially the former. And antibiotics cause it to act up terribly. I take up to 300 mg of B$_6$ per day, and up to 1,000 mg of magnesium. I can't say it works perfectly, but when this condition started I couldn't even use a pair of scissors without pain; now I've just a bit of stiffness sometimes, especially premenstrually. The alternatives are splinting, anti-inflammatory drugs or surgery, and none of these necessarily eliminates the problem permanently.

Part III

Helping Yourself

The body of this book explains what you can do to improve your own health and well-being and that of your family through good nutrition, with particular emphasis on how nutrition affects your fertility. You probably recognize that good nutrition is your own responsibility or you wouldn't be reading this book. In a world of fast food restaurants, processed foods, and even completely prepared meals available in the frozen foods section of your local supermarket, it may be a bit overwhelming. Therefore, I want to stress that you are not alone—whether your concern is just general nutrition or whether it is the desire to remedy some irregularity in your own fertility or a problem of mutual infertility. You can get help.

You may find that the information in this book is sufficient to put you on the right track, especially if any problems you have are minor ones. You can also get personal help from a nutritional counselor; you can get help from additional books, and you can get help from certain resource organizations. You are very definitely not alone.

15

Finding a Nutritional Counselor

Nutritional counseling is a basic component of health care involving nutrition for prevention or healing. The knowledge level of your nutritional advisor will certainly affect health decisions that you make, so selecting such an individual is not a casual undertaking. What, then, are the attributes that you should look for? Below are several traits that in my mind typify the ideal nutritional counselor. (Please note that while this person may be of either gender, I have used the pronoun "he" throughout to avoid cumbersome grammatical inventions.)

1. He is a qualified health professional, educated in the functions of the human body. He could be a medical doctor, an osteopathic doctor, a chiropractor, a nutritionist or one of the less familiar naturopathic or homeopathic doctors. For those with serious health problems such as cardiovascular disease or diabetes, every effort should be made to find a medical or osteopathic doctor who is aware of the benefits of nutrition for the particular condition.

2. He is enthusiastically interested in the role of nutrition in health and disease, and he stays informed about new research involving nutrition and health. This trait cannot be determined by the letters that follow a health professional's

name. To assume, for example, that a medical doctor cannot fit this description because "doctors don't learn about nutrition in medical school" is erroneous. It is equally erroneous to assume that a degree in any of the health professions automatically confers interest or expertise in nutrition on the recipient of that degree.

3. He does not restrict his own effectiveness by clinging to the belief that supplements are unnecessary if a "balanced diet" is eaten. You may be surprised to learn that this belief is held by a majority of those with formal training in nutrition. Patricia Hausman, a trained nutritionist with a distinguished career in the field, provides eye-opening insights into her profession:

Having a master's degree in nutrition, I know firsthand just how strongly my fellow nutritionists frown on supplement use. In fact, I have spent years trying to trace the origins of my profession's prejudice against vitamins and other supplements....

Like all university-educated nutritionists, I was taught to scorn supplements. It would have been impossible, I think, to complete my graduate degree in nutrition without having felt a constant pressure to decry their use. Rare was the nutrition textbook that didn't assail supplement use and equate it with "food faddism," an expression that I abhor. And the pressure to deplore supplement use continued after graduation, throughout my seven years at the Center for Science in the Public Interest [Washington, D.C.], and while writing my first two books.[1]

Like Patricia Hausman, there are other nutritionists, dietitians and nurses who have had similar training but whose experience with vitamin and mineral supplements has led them to re-evaluate and reject this aspect of their education. The combination of one of these backgrounds plus openness to supplementation can make for an excellent counselor.

4. He is not only open to your input; he considers your awareness and participation in your health care indispensable. He sees health care as an equal partnership with his

client, and he recognizes that ultimate decision-making rests with you. He asks you to read pamphlets and even whole books. He is unafraid to say, "I don't know," and he appreciates published information or anecdotes that you provide to help him help you more effectively.

5. He recognizes the role of the emotions in health and healing, and he is genuinely encouraging and uplifting about the healing power of the human body.

6. He is available by telephone. After an initial visit or two, he is prompt and gracious about answering your questions on the phone. He knows you're not made of money.

How do you find such an "ideal" nutritional counselor?

Rest assured that such individuals do exist (I selected the foregoing traits by reflecting on the attributes of four such individuals whom I have dealt with in our own medium-sized community). Such professionals are highly esteemed by the laymen who use their services, and locating their clients is the key to locating your nutritional counselor.

Food co-ops are often the unofficial clearinghouse for information on every variety of alternative health care, including the names and reputations of nutritionally-oriented medical doctors, osteopaths, chiropractors and so forth. Keep in mind that co-op employees are often members who work only a few hours per week, so if one person can't help you, perhaps the next day's employees can! Privately-owned health food stores may be equally helpful. At an excellent health food shop in my community, customers can readily obtain the names of physicians who regularly refer patients to the shop for supplements.

I personally was able to obtain the services of an excellent nutritional counselor, a chiropractor, by consulting the listing of chiropractors in the "Yellow Pages" of the telephone directory. The notation of his interest in nutritional counseling proved very useful. The advertising pages of the phone book may aid you in locating local nutritionists or even herbalists (try "Nutritionists," "Health Food," and "Herbs").

Two books may also aid the search for a counselor. *The Directory of Holistic Medicine and Alternative Health Care Services in the U.S.** contains over one thousand city-by-city listings of nutritionally-oriented medical doctors and many lesser-known health professionals. *The Yeast Syndrome** contains a large directory of medical doctors and osteopathic doctors who treat the disease candidiasis (yeast overgrowth). Since yeast overgrowth is treated with unrefined foods and supplements, as well as with drugs, it is likely that many of these physicians will also treat non-yeast diseases with emphasis on nutrition. Health professionals whom you contact via either of these two sources may also be able to refer you to a nutritional counselor closer to your home.

Can the doctor who is open but not especially knowledgeable about nutrition serve as an adequate nutritional counselor? The answer is a qualified "yes," in my opinion. If you have no serious health disorders, if you are willing to read in the field of nutrition, you may get along very well by simply letting your doctor know what you are doing. Your excellent health probably contributes to his openness to nutrition. On the other hand, you may have more to gain if you have the input of another nutritional advisor along with a supportive primary doctor. My experience is that this is a very workable situation as long as the doctor isn't "down on it because he's not up on it!"

Your health insurance plan could be a significant obstacle in your search for a nutritional counselor. Health maintenance organizations (HMOs) look attractive on the surface, but they restrict members to a list of participating providers. Traditional health insurance policies offer far more flexibility in allowing you to choose your own doctors. My recommendation for those who are interested in any form of alternative health care, including holistic nutrition, is to choose a traditional insurance plan if possible. It will give you financial access to a far greater number of health professionals than will the HMOs.

* See "Further Reading"

Further Reading

Berger, Stuart M., M.D. (1987). *How to Be Your Own Nutritionist.* New York: Avon Books. Excellent, up-to-date information on diet and supplements, and specific recommendations for many special cases. His protein allowances for pregnant women are far too low, in my opinion; other than that, I believe this is the best book on general nutrition currently available.

Berger, Stuart M., M.D. (1988). *What Your Doctor Didn't Learn in Medical School.* New York: Avon Books. Covers difficult-to-diagnose diseases such as hypothyroidism, PMS, hypoglycemia and candidiasis. Exceptionally helpful for those who feel unwell, yet are told by doctors that they "can find nothing wrong." Explains what tests are useful for accurately identifying these and other disorders.

Bricklin, Mark (1983). *The Practical Encyclopedia of Natural Healing.* Emmaus, PA: Rodale Press. Just as the title implies, this is a reference of nutritional or other natural cures. Includes a large variety of ailments, from acne, breech position and canker sores to varicose veins, warts and yeast infections. Even contains information on lupus, cystic fibrosis, multiple sclerosis and other serious disorders. Very chatty and easy to understand.

Crook, William G., M.D. (1986). *The Yeast Connection* (3rd ed.). New York: Vintage Books. This book is thoroughly documented and serves as the "bible" for the controversial disorder, candidiasis. Contains a questionnaire for determining the likelihood that you have yeast overgrowth. Has much information on environmental allergies also.

Davis, Adelle, revised by Marshall Mandell, M.D. (1981). *Let's Have Healthy Children.* New York: Signet Books. This book is an immense help both for pregnancy and for nutritional care of babies and children. Covers virtually every abnormality of pregnancy, with information aimed at preventing them. More a reference than a page-by-pager, but well worth digging into.

Ellis, John M., M.D., and Presley, James (1973). *Vitamin B₆: The Doctor's Report*. New York: Harper and Row. Chapter 7, "B₆ and Pregnancy," is essential reading for anyone concerned about preventing edema (swelling) and toxemia during pregnancy. If you have carpal tunnel syndrome, read chapters 1 and 4.

Gillespie, Larrian, M.D. (1986). *You Don't Have to Live With Cystitis!* New York: Avon Books. The moral tone of this book is frequently offensive, and I would prefer not to recommend it. However, it is simply outstanding in the contribution it makes to understanding the types of bladder diseases as well as the considerable role of diet and supplements in preventing or overcoming them. Will also help men with prostatitis.

Hausman, Patricia M. (1987). *The Right Dose*. New York: Ballantine Books. The most authoritative source for answering the question, "At what level is a vitamin or mineral supplement toxic?" Includes many references to scientific papers dealing with this subject. Inexplicably fails to cover iodine, which has a high potential for toxicity.

Johnson, Roberta Bishop, ed. (1981). *Whole Foods For the Whole Family*. Franklin Park, IL: La Leche League International. A lovely cookbook for those attempting to improve their home cooking. Uses all natural ingredients. Contains detailed sections on sprouting and bread baking, and even has a children's section. Many recipes offer options to accommodate allergic individuals, to improve nutrition or to add variety.

Kippley, Sheila (1989). *Breastfeeding and Natural Child Spacing: How Ecological Breastfeeding Spaces Babies* (2nd ed.). Cincinnati: Couple to Couple League. The very best book available on how to breastfeed, including long-term breastfeeding. Also the best information I know of on feeding solids during later babyhood. Sheila Kippley is the co-founder of the Couple to Couple League for Natural Family Planning. I am very grateful to her that I read the first edition of this book before my first child was born.

Kirschmann, John D. with Dunne, Lavon J. (1984). *Nutrition Almanac* (2nd ed.). New York: McGraw-Hill. *The* guide to prevention and healing through nutrition. Contains useful information on every vitamin and mineral, many charts of the nutrients found in particular foods, and even a section on herbs. Slightly out of date, but future editions are promised.

Linde, Shirley and Carrow, Donald J., M.D. (1985). *The Directory of Holistic Medicine and Alternative Health Care Services in the U.S.* Phoenix: Health Plus Publishers. Over a thousand city-by-city listings of nutritionally-aware health professionals, including medical doctors, osteopaths, chiropractors, homeopaths, naturopaths and dentists.

Mindell, Earl (1987). *Unsafe at Any Meal.* New York: Warner Books. If you have ever wondered exactly what is wrong with processed food, this registered pharmacist will explain it in laymen's terms. A great motivator for eating properly.

Prevention magazine editors (1984). *The Complete Book of Vitamins.* Emmaus, PA: Rodale Press. This book has highly useful information on a wide variety of disorders which may be helped with vitamins. The first few chapters make a strong case for the value of supplementation.

Shimmin, Delores (1984). *Health, Safety, and Manners 3.* Pensacola, FL: A Beka Book. A wonderful Christian health book with two chapters that heighten children's awareness of the value of good food and explain the role of nutrients in their bodies. Interest level: first through sixth grade; reading level: third through sixth grade. A must for homeschoolers.

Stout, Ruth and Clemence, Richard (1971). *The Ruth Stout No-Work Garden Book.* Emmaus, PA: Rodale Press. Describes the easiest way imaginable to garden organically. You need enough fall leaves, grass clippings, spoiled hay or straw to cover your garden deeply—and this book.

Trowbridge, John P., M.D., and Walker, Morton P., D.P.M. (1986). *The Yeast Syndrome.* New York: Bantam Books. Thick, carefully documented book on the controversial disorder, candidiasis. Very complete, including insight into the controversy surrounding yeast overgrowth and a directory of medical and osteopathic doctors who treat this disease.

Resources

The Couple to Couple League International
for Natural Family Planning
Box 111184
Cincinnati, Ohio 45211
Telephone: 513-661-7612

As a volunteer instructor for this organization, along with my husband, I am very partial to it. But I think that I am being completely objective to call it the world's best organization for learning the world's best method of birth control. CCL has over 700 teaching couples in the United States and in several foreign countries; find the ones nearest you by writing to the central office above.

The professionally trained teaching couples hold series of four monthly classes at local hospitals or churches. They cover all aspects of modern "sympto-thermal" natural family planning (NFP) including:

- health benefits of NFP
- effectiveness of NFP in preventing pregnancy; causes of surprise pregnancies
- NFP during breastfeeding and cycle irregularity
- achieving pregnancy through fertility awareness and other natural fertility aids
- NFP as a way of love and life.

Teaching couples also provide telephone counseling if cycle irregularities occur, and the method has built-in beginners' rules to help prevent surprise pregnancies among new users. A home study program is available for those who do not live in an area where the classes are taught. Whether you are having difficulty achieving pregnancy or are attempting to act in harmony with your body as you avoid a pregnancy, you will gain much from these interesting classes.

Mrs. Joy DeFelice
Director of Natural Family Planning Classes,
Educational Services Department
Sacred Heart Medical Center
West 101 Eighth Avenue, TAF-C9
Spokane, Washington 99220

If you would like more information concerning the role of night illumination in cycle irregularities, infertility or miscarriage, you may write to the above address. Enclose a stamped, self-addressed envelope.

Endometriosis Association
P. O. Box 92187
Milwaukee, WI 53202
Telephone: 1-800-992-ENDO (U.S.)
1-800-426-2END

This organization is an information exchange network for women with endometriosis. It promotes research on this disorder, maintains an information line, and sponsors local chapters which offer support and current information to interested women. Contact them at the above address or phone number for published material and referral to a chapter near you.

La Leche League International
9616 Minneapolis Avenue
Franklin Park, Illinois 60131
Telephone: 708-455-7730

Breastfeeding involves your baby's nutrition as well as your own. This wonderful organization is dedicated to helping mothers breastfeed successfully, no matter what adverse circumstances may be present. A series of four meetings is held at a leader's home to instruct and encourage you, and your leader provides non-medical telephone counseling also. By all means take the class *before* your baby is born if possible. You will also meet other like-minded mothers through "The League." If you cannot locate a League leader through your food co-op or white pages of the telephone directory, contact the central office above.

Madison Pharmacy Associates
429 Gammon Place
P. O. Box 9641
Madison, WI 53715
Telephone: 1-800-558-7046
in Wisconsin 1-800-362-7790

You can order Procycle, an excellent PMS supplement, through the above association. If you wish, you can arrange to have it mailed to you on a monthly basis, or you can order it by telephone as needed. Madison Pharmacy Associates is the parent organization of *PMS Access*.

NAPSAC International
Rt. 1, Box 646
Marble Hill, Missouri 63764
Telephone: 314-238-2010

NAPSAC stands for the (Inter)National Association of Parents and Professionals for Safe Alternatives in Childbirth. Their goals include promoting true natural childbirth, whether in home, hospital, or birthing center. They recognize the central role of nutrition to maternal and child health, and many of the books available through their book list focus on nutrition. There are NAPSAC member groups in twenty states and in Canada; their introductory packet of materials include names and addresses of these chapters. Their policies include a pro-life position.

PMS Access
P.O. Box 9326
Madison, WI 53715
Telephone: 1-800-222-4PMS
(in Wisconsin, 608-833-4PMS)

This organization serves as a clearinghouse for information and education concerning premenstrual syndrome (PMS). They maintain a referral list of physicians who treat PMS, and a catalogue of books, cassettes, articles and so forth about this disorder. Their bimonthly newsletter, *PMS Access*, contains timely articles on such topics as PMS and candidiasis, PMS and infertility, and PMS and tubal ligation. While you can subscribe to the newsletter for a modest cost, you will probably find it more useful to obtain their introductory materials and use their catalogue to select back issues of the newsletter which focus on the topics of particular interest to you. The chief focus of their information is nutrition, but they also cover pharmacological, psychological and other approaches to managing PMS. The toll-free number is for you to use if you have questions about PMS.

Radiance Products
A Division of American Health Plus Corporation
P. O. Box 119
Pearl River, NY 10965

Magna Natal is an excellent nonprescription prenatal multi-vitamin/multi-mineral manufactured by Radiance Products. I have no personal gain whatever in recommending one brand of supplement over another, but I find myself frequently suggesting this one to women who are preparing to conceive, women who are pregnant or breastfeeding, who are experiencing heavy bleeding or who are just plain fatigued for no apparent reason. It is also ideal for overcoming anemia. Because six tablets a day comprise the full dose, you can easily take less than the full dose and still maintain balance.

It is far better balanced and far more potent than prescription prenatal vitamins—I suggest that you compare the contents of the two. Women who use it during pregnancy are especially delighted with it. For example, one of our former infertility clients, who is soon expecting her sixth child at age thirty-seven—and meanwhile chauffering teenagers and mothering a toddler—says that she has had much more energy during her two "over thirty-five" pregnancies while taking Magna Natal than during her previous pregnancies throughout her twenties, when she used prescription prenatal vitamins.

If your local health food store does not carry Magna Natal, ask them to order it using the address above, or contact Radiance Products yourself.

References

Chapter 1: *Twelve Rules for Improved Nutrition*

1. Goei, G., M.D., J. Ralston, and G. Abraham, M.D., 1982. Dietary patterns of patients with premenstrual tension. J. Appl. Nutr. 34:9.
2. Kirschmann, J., with L. Dunne, 1984. Nutrition Almanac, 2nd ed., New York: McGraw-Hill, 93.

Chapter 5: *Premenstrual Syndrome*

1. Goei et al., 5.
2. Hargrove, J., M.D., and G. Abraham, M.D., 1983. The ubiquitousness of premenstrual tension in gynecologic practice. J. Reprod. Med. 28:435ff.
3. Abraham, G., M.D., 1983. Nutritional factors in the etiology of the premenstrual tension syndromes. J. Reprod. Med. 28:452.
4. Abraham, 1983, JRM, 452.
5. Dennefors, B., A. Sjogren, and L. Hamberger, 1982. Progesterone and adenosine 3', 5'-monophosphate formation by isolated human corpora lutea of different ages: Influence of human chorionic gonadotropin and prostaglandins. J. Clin. Endocrinol. Metab. 55:102ff.
6. Goldin, B., H. Adlercreutz, M.D., S. Gorbach, J. Warram, M.D., J. Dwyer, L. Swenson, and M. Woods, 1982. Estrogen excretion patterns and plasma levels in vegetarian and omnivorous women. N. Engl. J. Med. 307:1542ff.
7. Abraham, G., M.D., and R. Rumley, M.D., 1987. Role of nutrition in managing the premenstrual tension syndromes. J. Reprod. Med. 32:407.
8. Hargrove, J., M.D., and G. Abraham, M.D., 1979. Effect of vitamin B_6 on infertility in women with the premenstrual tension syndrome. Infertility 2:315ff.
9. Abraham, G., M.D., and J. Hargrove, M.D., 1980. Effect of vitamin B_6 on premenstrual symptomatology in women with premenstrual tension syndromes: A double blind crossover study. Infertility 3:155ff; Williams, M., R. Harris, and B. Dean, 1985. Controlled trial of pyridoxine in the premenstrual syndrome. J. Int. Med. Res. 13:174ff.
10. Abraham and Rumley, JRM, 405ff.
11. Abraham, 1983, JRM. 453-454.
12. Abraham, G., M.D., and M. Lubran, M.D., 1981. Serum and red cell magnesium levels in patients with premenstrual tension. Am. J. Clin. Nutr. 34:2364ff.
13. Goei, et al., 4ff.

14. Abraham, 1983, JRM, 458-459.
15. Goei, et al., 4ff.
16. Abraham, 1983, JRM, 455-456.
17. Abraham, G., M.D., 1984. Nutrition and the premenstrual tension syndromes. J. Appl. Nutr. 36:111.
18. Halbreich, U., M. Ben-David, M. Assael, and R. Bornstein, 1976. Serumprolactin in women with premenstrual syndrome. The Lancet, Sept. 25, 654ff.
19. Horrobin, D., 1983. The role of essential fatty acids and prostaglandins in the premenstrual syndrome. J. Reprod. Med. 28:465.
20. Horrobin, 465ff.
21. Horrobin, 465ff.
22. Kass-Annese, B., and H. Danzer, M.D., 1984. The Complete Guide to the Treatment of Premenstrual Problems. Santa Monica, CA: Patterns Publishing Co., 52.
23. Delitala, G., A. Masala, S. Alagna, and L. Devilla, 1976. Effect of pyridoxine on human hypophyseal trophic hormone release: A possible stimulation of hypothalamic dopaminergic pathway. J. Clin. Endocrinol. Metab. 42:603ff.
24. Abraham and Rumley, 412.
25. London, R., M.D., G. Sundaram, L. Murphy, and P. Goldstein, M.D., 1983. Evaluation and treatment of breast symptoms in patients with the premenstrual syndrome. J. Reprod. Med. 28:503ff.
26. Budoff, P., M.D., 1983. The use of prostaglandin inhibitors for the premenstrual syndrome. J. Reprod. Med. 28:469.
27. Minton, J., M.D., M. Foeking, D. Webster, and R. Matthews, 1979. Response of fibrocystic disease to caffeine withdrawal and correlation of cyclic nucleotides with breast disease. Am. J. Obstet. Gynecol. 135:157ff.
28. Abraham, 1983, JRM, 458.
29. Goei, G., M.D., and G. Abraham, M.D., 1983. Effect of a nutritional supplement, Optivite, on symptoms of premenstrual tension. J. Reprod. Med. 28:527ff.
30. Abraham and Rumley, 405ff.
31. Chakmakjian, Z., M.D., C. Higgins, and G. Abraham, M.D., 1985. The effect of a nutritional supplement, Optivite[R] for Women, on premenstrual tension syndromes: II. Effect on symptomatology, using a double blind cross-over design. J. Appl. Nutr. 37:12ff.
32. Abraham and Rumley, 413.
33. When vitamin B_6 has been taken at levels of 2,000 to 6,000 mg per day over a prolonged time period, serious neural dysfunction has occurred (Schaumburg, H., M.D., J. Kaplan, M.D., A. Windebank, M.D., N. Vick, M.D., S. Rasmus, M.D., D. Pleasure, M.D., and M. Brown, M.D., 1983. Sensory neuropathy from pyridoxine abuse. New England J. Med. 309:445ff.). This study has been confirmed, and three individuals taking vitamin B_6 at levels of 200 to 500 mg for a prolonged period developed this neural dysfunction also (Parry, F., and D. Bredesen, 1985. Sensory

neuropathy with low-dose pyridoxine. Neurology 35:1466ff.). Note that in all cases other vitamins and minerals were not reported to have been taken simultaneously (though the 2,000 mg doses of B_6 are indefensible under any circumstances).

34. Prevention editors, 1984. The Complete Book of Vitamins. Emmaus, PA: Rodale Press, 162-163; hereafter CBV.

35. Davis, A., revised by M. Mandell, M.D., 1981. Let's Have Healthy Children. New York: Signet Books, 299.

Chapter 6: *Cycle Irregularities and Female Infertility*

1. Bonaventura, L., M.D., personal communication, April 12, 1990.

2. Strott, C., C. Cargille, G. Ross, and M. Lipsett, 1970. The short luteal phase. J. Clin. Endocrol. 30:246ff.

3. Bonaventura, L., M.D., personal communication.

4. Corenblum, B., M.D., N. Pairaudeau, M.D., and A. Shewchuk, M.D., 1976. Prolactin hypersecretion and short luteal phase defects. Obstet. Gynecol. 47:487.

5. Seppala, M., E. Hirvonen, and T. Ranta, 1976. Hyperprolactinaemia and luteal insufficiency. The Lancet, January 31, 229ff.); Bahamondes, L., M.D., W. Saboya, M.D., M. Tambascia, M.D., and M. Trevisan, M.D., 1979. Galactorrhea, infertility, and short luteal phases in hyperprolactinemic women: Early stage of amenorrhea-galactorrhea? Fert. Steril. 32:476ff.; Kauppila, A., P. Leinonen, R. Vihko, and P. Ylostalo, 1982. Metoclopramide-induced hyperprolactinemia impairs ovarian follicle maturation and corpus luteum function in women. J. Clin. Endocrinol. Metab. 54:955ff.

6. McIntosh, E., 1976. Treatment of women with the galactorrhea-amenorrhea syndrome with pyridoxine (vitamin B_6). J. Clin. Endocrinol. Metab. 42:1192ff.

7. Abraham, 1983, 446ff.

8. Abraham and Rumley, 405ff.

9. Kass-Annese and Danzer, 65.

10. Hargrove and Abraham, 1979, 315ff.

11. Kass-Annese and Danzer, 66.

12. Bricklin, M., ed., 1986. The Natural Healing Annual. Emmaus, PA: Rodale Press, 151.

13. Melotte-Athmer, A., M.D., 1986. Iodine needed for proper thyroid function. The CCL News 12 (5):3.

14. Kirschmann and Dunne, 170.

15. Berger, S., M.D., 1988. What Your Doctor Didn't Learn In Medical School. New York: Avon Books, 103-104.

16. Berger, S., M.D., 1987. How To Be Your Own Nutritionist. New York: Avon Books, 341.

17. Bricklin, ed., 1986, 151-152.

18. Frisch, R., 1988. Fatness and fertility, Sci. Am., March, 92.

19. Frisch, 93.

20. "In underweight or excessively lean women the patterns of secretion of

gonadotropin-releasing hormone is abnormal in amount and timing and is similar to that of prepubertal girls." Frisch, 92.

21. Frisch, 91.
22. Women superdieters and runners may lose the fertility stakes. Medical World News, April 27, 1981, 27ff.
23. Frisch, 91.
24. Abraham and Rumley, 1987, 418.
25. Abraham, 1984, 107.
26. Wynn, V., 1975. Vitamins and oral contraceptive use. The Lancet, March 8, 561ff.
27. Prevention editors, 1984, 98-100.
28. Wilcox, A., C. Weinburg, and D. Baird, 1988. Caffeinated beverages and decreased fertility. The Lancet, December 24/31, 1453ff.
29. Christianson, R., F. Oechsli, and B. van den Berg, 1989. Caffeinated beverages and decreased fertility. The Lancet, February 18, 378.
30. DeFelice, J., 1985. The effects of light on cervical mucus patterns in the menstrual cycle: A clinical study. Available through Sacred Heart Medical Center, Spokane, WA.
31. J. DeFelice, personal communication.
32. DeFelice, 1985, 4.
33. DeFelice, personal communication.
34. DeFelice, 1985, 5.
35. DeFelice, 1985, 25.
36. DeFelice, 1985, 27.
37. Abraham, 1983, 453; Abraham and Rumley, 1987, 407.
38. Abraham, 1983, 453.
39. Labrum, A., 1983. Hypotholamic, pineal and pituitary factors in the premenstrual syndrome. J Reprod. Med. 28:441.
40. Wurtman, R., and Y. Ozaki, 1978. Physiological control of melatonin synthesis and secretion: Mechanisms generating rhythms in melatonin, methoxytryptophol, and arginine vasotocin levels and effects on the pineal of endogenous catecholamines, the estrous cycle, and environmental lighting. J. Neural. Transm. Suppl. 13:59.
41. Abraham, 1983, 453.
42. Muenter, M., H. Perry, and J. Ludwig, 1971. Chronic vitamin A intoxication in adults. Hepatic, neurologic and dermatologic complications. Am. J. Med. 50:129ff.
43. Kemmann, E., M.D., S. Pasquale, M.D., and R. Skaf, M.D., 1983. Amenorrhea associated with carotenemia. JAMA 249:926ff.

Chapter 7: *Difficult Menstruation*

1. Lithgow, D., and W. Politzer, 1977. Vitamin A in the treatment of menorrhagia. S. African Med. J. 51:191ff.
2. Hausman, P., 1987. The Right Dose. New York: Ballantine Books, 37.
3. Berger, 1987, 311.
4. CBV, 1984, 99.

5. Hausman, 348ff.
6. Horrobin, 466.
7. Abraham, 1983, 452.
8. Weller, S., 1987. Pain-Free Periods. Rochester, VT: Thorsons Publishers, Inc., 51.
9. "If... a major problem in PMS is defective formation of PGE_1 [prostaglandin E_1, a beneficial prostaglandin] ..., then NSAID [nonsteroid anti-inflammatory drugs], which will also block PGE_1 production, may actually aggravate some features of PMS." Horrobin, 466.
10. Endometriosis. PMS Access, May/June, 1988, 1-3.
11. Hargrove and Abraham, 1983, 436.
12. Hargrove, J., M.D., verbal communication, 6 April, 1990.
13. Kass-Annese and Danzer, 66.
14. Abraham and Rumley, 405ff.

Chapter 8: *Vaginal Infections*

1. Prevention editors, 1989. Medical Care Yearbook. Emmaus, PA: Rodale Press, 181; hereafter MCY.
2. MCY, 181.
3. MCY, 182.
4. Crook, W., M.D., 1986. The Yeast Connection, 3rd ed. New York: Vintage Books, 364.
5. Horowitz, B., M.D., S. Edelstein, M.D., and L. Lippman, M.D., 1984. Sugar chromatography studies in recurrent *Candida* vulvovaginitis. J. Reprod. Med. 29:441.
6. Trowbridge, J., M.D., and M. Walker, D.P.M., 1986. The Yeast Syndrome. New York: Bantam Books, 267.
7. Horowitz, B., M.D., S. Edelstein, M.D., and L. Lippman, M.D., 1987. Sexual transmission of Candida. Obstet. Gynecol. 69:883ff.
8. Horowitz et al., 884.
9. Trowbridge and Walker, 388-406.
10. MCY, 187.
11. MCY, 187, 191.
12. Berger, 1987, 155.
13. MCY, 187-188.
14. MCY, 188.

Chapter 9: *Pregnancy*

1. Ellis, J., M.D., and J. Presley, 1973. Vitamin B_6: The Doctor's Report. New York: Harper and Row, 90, 96-97.
2. Ellis and Presley, 112-113.
3. Ellis and Presley, 113.

Chapter 10: *Repeated Miscarriages and Birth Defects*

1. Bahamondes et al., 476; Corenblum et al., 486.
2. Strott et al., 246ff.

3. DeFelice, 27.
4. Davis and Mandell, 20-21.
5. Davis and Mandell, 22-23.
6. CBV, 311.
7. Smithells, R., S. Sheppard, C. Schorah, M. Seller, N. Nevin, R. Harris, A. Read, and D. Fielding, 1980. Possible prevention of neural-tube defects by periconceptional vitamin supplementation. The Lancet, Feb. 16, 339ff.
8. Smithells, R., M. Seller, R. Harris, D. Fielding, C. Schorah, N. Nevin, S. Sheppard, A. Read, S. Walker and J. Wild, 1983. Further experience of vitamin supplementation for prevention of neural tube defect recurrences. The Lancet, May 7, 1027ff; Laurence, K., N. James, M. Miller, G. Tennant, and H. Campbell, 1981. Double-blind randomised controlled trial of folate treatment before conception to prevent recurrence of neural-tube defects. Br. Med. J. 282:1509ff.
9. Laurence, K., N. James, M. Miller, and H. Campbell, 1980. Increased risk of recurrence of pregnancies complicated by fetal neural tube defects in mothers receiving poor diets, and possible benefit of dietary counselling. Br. Med. J. 281:1592ff; Laurence, K., 1983. Dietary approaches to the prevention of neural tube defects. Nutrition and Health 2:181ff.
10. Mulinare, J., M.D., J. Cordero, M.D., J. Erickson, and R. Berry, M.D., 1988. Periconceptional use of multivitamins and the occurrence of neural tube defects. JAMA 260:3141ff.
11. Milunsky, A., H. Jick, M.D., S. Jick, C. Bruell, D. Mac Laughlin, K. Rothman, and W. Willet, M.D., 1989. Multivitamin/folic acid supplementation in early pregnancy reduces the prevalence of neural tube defects. JAMA 262:2847ff.
12. Tolarova, M., 1982. Periconceptional supplementation with vitamins and folic acid to prevent recurrence of cleft lip. The Lancet, July 24, 217.
13. Davis and Mandell, 25.
14. Davis and Mandel, 24.
15. Hausman, 39.
16. Manson, J., and R. Simons. Influence of environmental agents on male reproductive failure. In Hunt, V., 1979. Work and the Health of Women. Boca Raton, FL: CRC Press, 174.
17. Manson and Simons, 155.
18. Weathersbee, P., 1980. Early reproductive loss and the factors that may influence its occurrence. J. Reprod. Med. 25:316.

Chapter 11: *The Premenopause*

1. Berger, 1987, 155.
2. Hargrove and Abraham, 1983, 436-437.
3. Kass-Annese and Danzer, 67.
4. Kass-Annese and Danzer, 67-68.
5. Frisch, 92.
6. Kass-Annese and Danzer, 67.
7. Mendelsohn, R., M.D., 1981. Male Practice: How Doctors Manipulate Women. Chicago, IL: Contemporary Books, 91.

8. Zussman, L., M.D., S. Zussman, R. Sunley, and E. Bjornson, 1981. Sexual response after hysterectomy-oophorectomy: Recent studies and reconsideration of psychogenesis. Am. J. Obstet. Gynecol. 140:725ff.

9. Zussman et al., 727.

10. Gillespie, L., M.D., 1986. You Don't Have to Live With Cystitis! New York: Avon Books, 178ff.

Chapter 12: *The Male Connection*

1. Guyton, A., M.D., 1984. Textbook of Medical Physiology, 6th ed., Philadelphia: W.B. Saunders Co., 995.

2. Harris, W., T. Harden, and E. Dawson, 1979. Apparent effect of ascorbic acid medication on semen metal levels. Fert. Steril. 32:456-457.

3. Harris et al., 457.

4. Dawson, E., W. Harris, W. Rankin, L. Charpentier, and W. McGanity, 1987. Effect of ascorbic acid on male fertility. Ann. New York Acad. Sci. 498:312ff.

5. Dawson et al, 320.

6. Dawson et al, 321.

7. Gonzalez, E., 1983. Sperm swim singly after vitamin C therapy. JAMA 249:2747.

8. Prasad, A., 1985. Clinical, endocrinologic, and biochemical effects of zinc deficiency. Spec. Topics in Endocrinol. Metab. 7:59-60.

9. Prasad, 69.

10. Hartoma, T., K. Nahoul, and A. Netter, 1977. Zinc, plasma androgens and male sterility. The Lancet, Sept. 26, 1125-1126.

11. Calloway, D., 1983. Nutrition and reproductive function of men. Nutrition Abstracts and Reviews/Reviews in Clinical Nutrition 53:373.

12. Calloway, 375.

13. Calloway, 369.

14. Wu, S., J. Oldfield, P. Whanger, and P. Weswig, 1973. Effect of selenium, vitamin E, and antioxidants on testicular function in rats. Biol. Reprod. 8:625ff.

15. Berger, 1987, 310-312.

16. Berger, 1987, 143.

17. Berger, 1987, 231.

18. Berger, 1987, 345.

19. Weathersbee, 316.

20. Weathersbee, P., and J. Lodge, 1978. A review of ethanol's effects on the reproductive process. J. Reprod. Med. 21:63.

21. Weathersbee, P., and J. Lodge, 1977. Caffeine: Its direct and indirect influence on reproduction. J. Reprod. Med. 19:60.

22. Weathersbee and Lodge, 1977, 60.

23. Prasad, 59-60.

24. Stogdill, B., M.D., July, 1989, verbal communication.

25. Berger, 1987, 143.

26. Berger, 1987, 311, 324.

Chapter 13: *Candidiasis*

1. Crook, The Yeast Connection, page 1 of introductory section titled "What This Book is All About."
2. Crook, 181-182.
3. Trowbridge and Walker, 127-128.
4. PMS and Candida albicans yeast theory. PMS Access, Nov/Dec., 1986, 1-2.
5. Trowbridge and Walker, 187.
6. Galland, L., M.D., 1986. Nutrition and Candida albicans. In Bland, J., 1986. A Year in Nutritional Medicine, 2nd ed. New Canaan, CT: Keats Publishing, Inc., 211-220.
7. Crook, 369; Trowbridge and Walker, 168-169.
8. Trowbridge and Walker, 165-166.

Chapter 14: *Questions and Answers*

1. Kapcala, L., M.D., 1984. Galactorrhea and thyrotoxicosis. Arch. Intern. Med. 144:2349ff.
2. McIntosh, 1192ff.
3. Kapcala, 2350.
4. Bricklin, M., 1983. The Practical Encyclopedia of Natural Healing. Emmaus, PA: Rodale Press, 499-502.
5. Gillespie, 244.
6. Gillespie, 253-256.
7. Abraham and Rumley, 406-407.
8. Abraham, 1984, 111.
9. Wolaniuk, A., S. Vadhanavkit, and K. Folkers, 1983. Electromyographic data differentiate patients with the carpal tunnel syndrome when double blindly treated with pyridoxine and placebo. Res. Commun. Chem. Pathol. Pharmacol. 41:501.

Chapter 15: *Finding a Nutritional Counselor*

1. Hausman, 4, 8.

Index

feine, 51, 129; problems, and sugar consumption, 128, 129; tenderness, as symptom of PMS, 47; tenderness, decreased by vitamin E, 51

Breast milk (See "Milk, mother's.")

Breastfeeding (nursing), and babies' nutrition, 17, 38; and breast cancer, 132; breast fullness unrelated to, 129; as cause of cycle irregularities, 126; effect on female fertility, 57-59; and endometriosis, 81; further information on, 141, 144, 146; minimum daily food goals during, 96-97 (Table 7); among NFP users, 1; night lighting recommendations during, 71

Breastfeeding and Natural Child Spacing, 17, 141

Bromocriptine (Parlodel), 129

Bulimia, 65

Butter, compared with margarine, 36

C

Caffeine (See also "Coffee."), and anxiety, 38; and breast problems, 51, 128, 129; consumption and PMS, 51; consumption, before conception, 100-101; and cycle irregularity or infertility, 68-69, 115, 127; decreasing consumption of, 36-37; and hypoglycemia, 9, 12, 50; and male fertility, 115; and migraine headaches, 95, 132; and miscarriage, related to male animal intake of, 104; during weight loss, 67; and vaginal yeast infections, 86-87

Calcium (See also "Calcium-magnesium ratio."), balance with magnesium, 31, 38, 79, 81; for blood clotting and heavy bleeding, 79; for menstrual pain, 81; in Optivite, 55 (Table 6); and osteoporosis, 108, 133; in Shaklee Vita-C, 113; suggested daily supplement, 33 (Table 5); and vitamin D, 31, 79

Calcium-magnesium ratio, in dairy products, 49; effect on insulin, 50; after menopause, 108; for menstrual pain, 83; in Optivite and Procycle, 52; for PMS, 53; to prevent osteoporosis, 133

Calories, during pregnancy, 94, 95

Candida albicans, in vaginal infections, 85-86; and candidiasis, 119

Candidiasis, 119-123; as cause of PMS-like symptoms, 54; and cycle irregularity and female infertility, 73; doctors who treat, 139, 142; further reading on, 140, 142, 145; nutrition for, 121-122; and Pill use, 67; predisposing factors, 120; and prostatitis, 118, 120, 122; symptoms of, 119-120; and vaginal yeast infections, 87-88

Capsicum (See "Cayenne pepper tablets.")

Carbohydrates, complex, defined and recommended, 5; to overcome hypoglycemia, 16, 69, 132; as part of evening meal, 15-16; in PMS diet, 52; to prevent migraines, 132

Carotene, beta, and candidiasis, 121; dietary sources of, 78; excessive, effects on cycle, 73; for heavy, prolonged menses, 78

Carpal tunnel syndrome (See also "Hand symptoms."), 133-134; further reading, 141

Cayenne pepper tablets (capsicum), for heavy bleeding, 79, 80

Childbirth at home, 93-94; further information on, 145

Chlorophyll, for blood clotting, heavy menses, and postpartum bleeding, 79

Chromium, depleted by sugar, 9; to maintain blood glucose levels, 50; in Optivite, 55 (Table 6); suggested daily supplement, 33 (Table 5)

Cis-linoleic acid (See also "Linoleic acid."), as precursor of prostaglandin E_1, 49; -containing foods in PMS diet, 52

Cleft lip (See also "Birth defects."), and folic acid, 103

Clomid (See also "Fertility drugs."), inadvisability of, if underweight, 65

Clotting, blood, and menstrual bleeding, 78-79

Coffee (See also "Caffeine."), 6; and bladder infections, 130; and breast problems, 51, 129; and cycle irregularity and infertility, 68-69, 127; and male fertility, 115; and migraine headache, 132; and PMS, 51; and prostatitis, 117; as source of caffeine, 12

Confusion, as symptom of PMS, 48

Constipation, as symptom of candidiasis, 119; and prostatitis, 117

Contraceptives, oral (See "Birth control pills.")

Copper, for anemia, 80; balance with zinc, 31; in Optivite, 55 (Table 6); suggested daily supplement, 33 (Table 5)

Corpus luteum (See also "Luteal phase."), abnormal function of in PMS, 48-49; and elevated estrogen, 66; function of, 44; function and vitamin B_6, 61; and miscarriage, 100; and PMS nutritional plan, 48-49, 82, 100; and preovulatory events, 5

Corticosteroids, and candidiasis, 120

Counseling, nutritional, 136-139; after discontinuing Pill, 68; for galactorrhea, 129; for heavy menstruation, 79, 80; recommended, 3; for sensitivity to night lighting, 72; when supplementing, 30

Counselor, nutritional, 38, 135-139

Country Journal, 23

Couple to Couple League for Natural Family Planning 2, 43, 62, 73, 74, 75, 86, 88, 115, 133, 141; further information on, 143

Cramps, menstrual (See "Menstruation, painful.")

Craving for sweets, overcoming, 36-37; as symptom of hypoglycemia, 49; as symptom of PMS, 48

Crook, William, M.D., 122, 123, 140

Crying, as symptom of PMS, 48

Cycle irregularities, 57-73; and birth control pills, 67-68, 127; and breastfeeding, 57-58, 126; and caffeine consumption, 68-69, 127; checklist of possible causes of, 125-128; and dieting, ix, 64-65, 127; and exercise ix-x, 65, 127; and hyperthyroidism, 62-63; improved

100-101; specialist for, 75-76; and underweight, 63-65

Infertility, female, secondary, overcome after caffeine reduction, 68; overcome with vitamin B$_6$, 61; PMS nutritional plan for, 61; related to underweight, 65

Infertility, male, 111-116; factors contributing to, 115; nutrients to overcome, 112-115; and sperm count, 112; and spermagglutination, 112, 113; and wife's role, 115-116

Insomnia (See also "Sleep disruption."), as symptom of PMS, 48

Insulin, and caffeine consumption, 12; overproduction, 9, 50; in PMS, 50

Insurance, health, 139

Intrauterine devices (IUDs), and vaginal infections, 86, 88

Intercourse, sexual, and bladder infection, 129-130; frequency of, and zinc, 113; and hysterectomy, 109; inadvisability during vaginal infections, 87, 89; increased frequency of, for prostatitis, 116-117; irritation during, as symptom of bacterial vaginal infection, 88; pain during, as symptom of endometriosis, 81; pain during, as symptom of prostatitis, 116; and sperm quantity, 112; timing of, to achieve pregnancy, 2, 75

Iodine, for cycle irregularities of breastfeeding, 126; for cycle irregularities or infertility, 61-62, 128; in kelp tablets, ix, 62; maximum recommended dose of, 62; to prevent miscarriage, 101; in Optivite, 55 (Table 6); overdose, related to hyperthyroidism, 63; RDA for, 62; suggested daily supplement, 33 (Table 5); and thyroid function ix, 61-63; toxicity of, 33, 62, 141

Iron, destroys vitamin E, 101; levels lowered by aspirin, 27; in Magna Natal, 80; in Optivite, 55 (Table 6); suggested daily supplement, 33 (Table 5); toxicity of, 33, 80

Irregular cycles (See "Cycle irregularities.")

Irregular shedding (See also "Spotting."), and luteal phase deficiency, 58

Irritability, and caffeine consumption, 12; and calcium supplements, 108; and hypoglycemia, 9; improved by evening primrose oil, 50; during Pill use, 67; as symptom of PMS, 47

Irritation or dryness, vaginal, causes of, 86, 88; in pre- or postmenopausal women, 89, 107-108

K

Kasse-Annese, Barbara, 61

Kelp, as source of iodine, ix, 62, 63

Kippley, Sheila, 17, 141

L

Lactation, 5 (See also "Breastfeeding.")

La Leche League International 2, 24; further information on, 144

Let's Have Healthy Children, 95, 101, 140

Linoleic acid (See also "Cis-linoleic acid."), 5, 6; for male fertility, 114

Low birth weight, and calorie and protein intake of mother, 94

Luteal phase, defined, 44; hormonal profile and breast cancer, 132; inadequacy, in cycle irregularity or infertility, 58-61; inadequacy, and PMS, 48-49; short, defined, 58; short, and galactorrhea, 128-129; short, and night lighting, 69-71; short, PMS nutritional plan for 47, 60, 127

Luteinizing hormone (LH), and amenorrhea, 58; and B vitamins, 114; and infertility, 59; inhibited by prolactin, 59; and normal ovulation, 43; and repeated miscarriage, 100; and sperm production, 112; in underweight women, 64

M

Madison Pharmacy Associates, 52, 145

Magna Natal, during breastfeeding, 126, 146; as general supplement, 39; for heavy, prolonged bleeding, 80, 146; micronutrient amounts in, 80, 93-94; ordering information, 146; for pregnancy 93-94, 146

Magnesium (See also "Calcium-magnesium ratio."), additional, 31; balance with calcium, 31, 79; for candidiasis, 121; for carpal tunnel syndrome, 134; depleted by sugar, 9; for galactorrhea, 128-129; link to night lighting, 71; in Magna Natal, 93-94; after menopause, 108; in millet, 36; for morning sickness, 131; in Optivite, 55 (Table 6); for painful menstruation, 81, 83; in PMS, 49, 50, 52, 53; during pregnancy, 93; in prescription prenatal vitamins, 95; to prevent osteoporosis, 133; in Shaklee Vita-C, 113; suggested daily supplement, 33 (Table 5); for yeast infections, 86

Male hormones (See "Androgens" and "Testosterone.")

Mandell, Marshall, M.D., 103, 142

Manganese, depleted by sugar, 9; in Optivite, 55 (Table 5); in Shaklee Vita-C, 113; suggested daily supplement, 33 (Table 5)

Margarine, compared with butter, 36; as source of saturated fat, 6, 49

"Mask" of pregnancy, 95

McIntosh, E. N., 129

Mendelsohn, Robert, M.D., 108-109

Menopause, 107-109 (See also "Premenopause."); amenorrhea of, 59; vaginal dryness after, 89

Menorrhagia (See "Menstruation, heavy or prolonged.")

Menses (See "Menstruation.")

Menstrual periods (See "Menstruation.")

Menstruation, and anorexia nervosa, 64; in anovulatory cycles, 58; cessation of, 107; lack of, 58; in long cycles, 77-78; loss of, in short cycles, 78; typical, defined, 77; and vaginal infection, 88

—heavy or prolonged, 77-80; after discontinuing Pill, 67, 78; hysterectomy for, 109; and NFP, ix, 2; and night lighting,

71; during premenopause, 107; as symptom of endometriosis, 81; as symptom of low thyroid function, 61, 78
—painful, 81-83; and endometriosis 73, 81-83; magnesium for, 81, 83; PMS nutritional plan for, 81
—scant, and excess vitamin A or carotene, 73; during Pill use, 78; as symptom of hyperthyroidism, 62
Midol, as source of caffeine, 12
Milk (See also "Dairy products.") 7, 15, 16, 108, 10 (Table 4), 96 (Table 7); allergy, 79; in breasts of non-nursing women, 60, 128; protein content of, 52
Milk, mother's, 9, 18, 38; as source of gamma-linoleic acid, 50
Minerals, chelated, 32
Minimum Daily Food Goals, (Table 4), 10-11
Minimum Daily Food Goals for Pregnant and Nursing Women (Table 7), 96-97
Miscarriage, early, caused by insufficient hormones, 59, 99-100; early, related to night lighting, 71, 100; father's role in preventing, 104-105; night lighting recommendations after, 71, 144; repeated, 99-101, 104-105
Mood swings, as symptom of PMS, 47
Moodiness, and food supplements, 39
Morning sickness (nausea), 130-131; prolonged, 93, 94
Mother Earth News, The, 23
Motrin, for painful menses, 81
Mucus, cervical, affected by estrogen and progesterone, 43, 44; affected by medicines, 73; during cycle irregularity and infertility, 58-59; extended, checklist of causes of, 126-128; lack of "more fertile," and vitamin A, 73; and male subfertility, 116; and NFP, ix, 44; PMS nutritional plan for scant or extended, 60; problems, related to overweight, 66; prolonged, as symptom of low thyroid function, 61, 62; scant, patchy, prolonged or ambiguous, and night lighting 69-71, 127; and vaginal infections, 73, 85, 88, 89
Muscle symptoms, related to candidiasis, 119

N

Natural family planning (NFP), based on fertility-menstrual cycle, 44; classes, 78; compared with holistic nutrition, 1-3; Couple to Couple League classes for, 143; and cycle irregularities ix-x, 2, 125-128; and vaginal infections, 85, 88
Natural foods, defined, 20; food co-op as source, 21; storage of, 12-13, 23-24
Nausea (See "Morning sickness.")
Nervous system symptoms, related to candidiasis, 119
Nervousness, 108 (See also "Anxiety" and "Irritability.")
Neural tube defects (See also "Birth defects."),

and folic acid, 102-103
Nicotine (See also "Smoking, cigarette."); before conception, 101; and male infertility, 115
Night lighting, sensitivity to (See "Sensitivity to night lighting.")
Nonsteroid anti-inflammatory drugs, 81
Numbness and tingling (See also "Hand symptoms."), and carpal tunnel syndrome, 133-134; during pregnancy, 93; as symptom of candidiasis, 119
Nursing (See "Breastfeeding.")
Nutrition Almanac, 28, 30, 42, 52, 94, 141-142
Nystatin, 121

O

Obesity (See "Overweight.")
Oil, dietary (See also "Fat, dietary."), fish, for candidiasis, 121; flaxseed, for candidiasis, 121; monounsaturated, 6, 11 (Table 4), 35, 97 (Table 7); needed for prostaglandin E_1 synthesis, 50; in PMS, 49, 50, 71; in PMS diet, 52; polyunsaturated, 5, 6, 11 (Table 4), 35, 97 (Table 7); unsaturated, 5, 7, 11 (Table 4), 35, 97 (Table 7); unsaturated, and prostate, 117; unsaturated, refrigeration of, 13; vegetable, 21-24;
Optivite, 39, 125; contents of, 55 (Table 6); for PMS, 52-53
Optivite, 12 Tablets (Table 6), 55
Oral contraceptives (See "Birth control pills.")
Oral-genital contact, and herpes simplex, 88-89; and urinary tract infections, 130; and vaginal bacterial infections, 88; and yeast infections, 87
Organic foods, defined, 20; sources of, 20-23
Organic Gardening, 23
Osteoporosis, 108, 133
Ovaries, function in normal fertility cycle, 43-45; after menopause, 107; removal of, and sexual desire, 109; restoration of function after Pill use, 67
Overdose (See also "Toxicity, vitamin or mineral."), micronutrient, 30; iodine, 63; vitamin A or carotene, 73
Overweight, and breast cancer, 132; and cycle irregularities or female infertility, 65-67, 127; and miscarriage, 100-101
Ovulation, in breastfeeding, cycle irregularity or infertility, 57-59;
—delayed, caused by underweight or dieting, 64; and dieting, ix; after discontinuing Pill, 67; caused by exercise, ix, 65; and low thyroid function, 127; and NFP, ix, 126-128; in nursing mother or cycle irregularities, 58; from stress, 76
—and miscarriage 99-100; normal, 43-45
—and role of sperm quantity, 112
Ovulation, medically induced (See "Fertility drugs.")
Ovum ("egg"), (See also "Ovulation."), immature, 58, 100; mature, 59; in normal fertility cycle, 43; and sperm, 111, 112

P

Pain, abdominal, and candidiasis, 119; breast, 51, 129 (See also "Breast."); in hands and arms, 92, 133-134; during intercourse, 116; between legs, rectal, or urethal, and prostatitis, 116; low back, and vaginal infection, 88; menstrual, 73, 77, 81-83, 119; muscle, and candidiasis, 119

Pantothenic acid, and birth defects, 103; for hay fever and colds, 73; and male fertility, 114; in Optivite, 55 (Table 6); suggested daily supplement, 32 (Table 5)

Parlodel (bromocriptine), 129

Penis, bacterial infection of, 89; yeast infection of, 87

Pergonal, 65 (See also "Fertility drugs.")

Period, menstrual (See "Menstruation.")

Physician's Reference to Natural Family Planning, A, 43

Pill, birth control (See "Birth control pills.")

Pineal gland, involved in light-dark rhythms, 69-70; and serotonin, 71-72

PMS Access, 2, 54; further information, 145

PMS, (See "Premenstrual syndrome [PMS].")

PMS diet, outlined, 51-52

PMS nutritional plan, for breast problems, 129; for cycle irregularities of unknown cause, 128; after discontinuing Pill, 67; for early miscarriage, 100; effect on prostaglandins, 81; effect on reproductive hormones, 47, 48-49, 60, 82, 100, 108; for endometriosis, 82-83; for luteal phase inadequacy, 60; for other disorders, 47; outlined, 51-53; for painful menses, 81, 83; during premenopause, 47, 108; for sensitivity to night lighting, 72

PMS supplements (See also "PMS nutritional plan."), 52-55, 125, 147

PMT-A (premenstrual tension-anxiety), defined, 47

PMT-C (premenstrual tension-carbohydrate craving), causes of, 49; defined, 48; and vitamin E, 51

PMT-D (premenstrual tension-depression), defined, 48; and vitamin E, 51

PMT-H (premenstrual tension-hyperhydration), defined, 47

Polysystemic chronic candidiasis (See "Candidiasis.")

Potassium, to maintain blood glucose levels, 50; in Optivite, 55; suggested daily supplement, 33

Potency, male, 113, 116

Pre-eclampsia (See "Toxemia of pregnancy.")

Pregnancy (conception) (See also "Pregnancy, achieving.") 91-97; clinical, and short luteal phase, 58; early, and birth defects, 99-100, 102-103; eclampsia of, 91-92; and endometriosis, 81; further reading, 141; and galactorrhea, 128; Magna Natal during, 93-94, 126, 146; male factors affecting, 104; minimum daily food goals during, 96-97 (Table 7); and morning sickness, 93, 94, 130-131; multiple, 38, 104, 120; nutritional needs during, 5, 27, 91-97; and PMS, 61; postponing or avoiding with NFP, ix, 125-128, 143; protein needs during, 94; and repeated miscarriage, 100-101; spotting during, 101; toxemia of, 91-93; and vaginal yeast infection, 86; weight gain during, 94

Pregnancy, achieving (See also "Infertility, female."), achieved through natural techniques, 74-75; achieved after night lighting adjustment, 70; achieved after thyroid medication reduction, 63; achieved with vitamin B_6 therapy, 60-61; achieved with vitamin C therapy in husband, 113; achieved after weight gain in underweight, 64; achieved after weight loss in overweight, 66; achievement while breastfeeding, 58-59; achievement delayed by caffeine, 68; Couple to Couple League classes for achieving or postponing, 143; fertility drugs and achieving, 59, 65, 66; fertility specialist for achieving, 75-76; luteal events if not achieved, 44; seeking, and NFP, ix, xi

Premature infants, and calorie and protein intake during pregnancy, 94; and folic acid, 101

Premenopause, 107-109, defined, 107; and hysterectomy, 108-109; and osteoporosis, 108; pattern of reduced fertility, 59, 127; PMS nutritional plan for 47, 108, 127; symptoms, 47, 107-108; and vaginal dryness, 108

Premenstrual syndrome (PMS) (See also "PMS nutritional plan."), 47-55; and abnormal fluid retention, 49-50; and abnormal luteal function, 48-49, 71; benefited by fertility observations, 44; and breast cancer, 132; and caffeine consumption, 51; and candidiasis, 119, 120; diet for, 51-52; effect on natural family planning, 2; and elevated prolactin levels, 50-51; and endometriosis, 82; further information, 140, 145-146; and nonsteroid anti-inflammatory drugs, 81, 151; and Optivite or Procycle, 52, 53, 125; and painful menses, 81, 83; related to other disorders, 3, 47; and serotonin, 71; supplements for, 52-53, 55 (Table 6); and vitamin E deficiency, 51

Premenstrual tension (PMT) (See "Premenstrual syndrome [PMS].")

Prenatal vitamins, prescription, inadequacy of, 95, 146; low potency of, 31; toxemia while taking, 91

Procycle, 39, 52, 125; ordering information, 145

Progesterone, and breast cancer, 132; effect on basal temperature, 44; effect on cervical mucus, 44; inhibited by prolactin, 59; levels increased by PMS nutritional plan, 48-49, 60, 82, 100, 132; levels increased by vitamin B_6, 61; low levels in PMS, 48; and miscarriage, 100; normal function of, 44; relation to endometriosis, 82; synthetic, and can-

riosis, 82; for galactorrhea, 128-129; and hand symptoms, 92, 93, 94, 95, 133-134; inadequacy of RDA during pregnancy, 95; inadequate in prescription prenatal vitamins, 95; in Magna Natal 93-94; for morning sickness, 131; nutritional counseling for, 32, 53; in Optivite, 55 (Table 6); in Optivite and Procycle, 52; for overcoming infertility in women with PMS, 60-61; for PMS, 53; for pregnancy edema, toxemia and eclampsia, 92-93; for prostaglandin E₁ synthesis, 49; for prostatitis, 117; suggested daily supplement, 32 (Table 5); and testes, 114; toxicity of, 32, 53, 148-149; for yeast infections, 86

Vitamin B₆:The Doctor's Report, 92, 141

Vitamin B₁₂, for anemia, 80; deficiency masked by folic acid, 31, 32; depleted by birth control pills, 67; and male fertility, 114; in Optivite, 32 (Table 6); suggested daily supplement, 32 (Table 5)

Vitamin C (ascorbic acid), additional, 31; for anemia, 80; for carpal tunnel syndrome, 134; depleted by birth control pills, 67; to eliminate toxins, 104; harmed by cooking, 7; for hay fever and colds, 73; levels lowered by aspirin, 27; and male fertility, 114; in Optivite, 55 (Table 6); for PMS, 53; to prevent miscarriage, 101; for prostaglandin E₁ synthesis, 49; for spermagglutination, 112-113, 115; suggested daily supplement, 32 (Table 5); for thyroid function, 62; for urinary tract infections, 130

Vitamin D, to absorb calcium, 31, 79, 133; for heavy or prolonged menstruation, 79; in Optivite, 55 (Table 6); and osteoporosis, 108, 133; for painful menses, 81; suggested daily supplement, 32 (Table 5)

Vitamin E, additional, 31; for anemia, 80; and birth defects, 103; for breast problems, 51, 128, 129; for cycle irregularities during breastfeeding, 126; for cycle irregularities of unknown cause, 128; deficiency as cause of PMS, 51; after discontinuing Pill, 67; to eliminate toxins, 104; harmed by cooking, 7; for hot flashes, 107-108; to increase energy, 38; and male fertility, 114; for normal menstruation, 78; in Optivite, 55 (Table 6); for PMT-C and PMT-D, 51; for preventing miscarriage, 101; for prostatitis, 117; and selenium, 31; suggested daily supplement, 32 (Table 5); for thyroid function, 62; for vaginal dryness, 89, 108; and vitamin A, 31, 73, 78, 103

Vitamin K, and "friendly bacteria", 79; dietary sources of, 79; for heavy menstruation, 78-79; levels lowered by aspirin, 27

Vitamins, timed-release, 32

W

Walker, Morton P., D.P.M., 123, 142

Water, drinking, for bladder infections, 130; chlorinated, and intestinal bacteria, 79;

purified sources of 13-14

Weight, body (See also "Overweight" and "Underweight."), before conception, 100-101; control of to achieve pregnancy, 74, 75; and cycle irregularity or infertility, x, 63-67, 127, 128; gain at menopause, 108; gain during pregnancy, 94; and PMS, 54

Weight loss, as cause of amenorrhea, 64-65; to improve fertility in overweight women, 66-67; as symptom of hyperthyroidism, 63

Weight to height ratio, role in female fertility, 63-65

What Your Doctor Didn't Learn in Medical School, 123, 140

Whole Foods for the Whole Family, 24, 141

Y

Yeast (See also "Candidiasis."), allergy, 122; brewer's, 80; infection, 85-88, 89;
—overgrowth, 119-123; further reading, 140, 142; and Pill use, 67; and prostatitis, 118; and reproductive disorders, 73; and yeast infections, 87-88;
—rapid action, 24

"Yeast-aware" doctors, how to locate, 87-88, 121

Yeast Connection, The, 122, 123, 140

Yeast Syndrome, The, 87, 121, 123, 139, 142

Yogurt, for candidiasis, 121; during antibiotic treatment, 86; as dairy food, 10 (Table 4), 96 (Table 7); douche, for vaginal yeast infections, 87; as food to emphasize, 7 (Table 2); making, 24; for meals or snacks, 15, 16; for prostatitis, 122; as source of intestinal bacteria, 79

You Don't Have to Live With Cystitis!, 109, 130, 142

Z

Zinc, balance with copper, 31, 33; depleted by sugar, 9; effect on prolactin, 51; and infertility, 33; lozenges for preventing colds, 73; and male fertility, 113, 114; and male potency and sexual desire, 113, 116; in Optivite, 55 (Table 6); to prevent birth defects, 103; to prevent miscarriage, 101; for prostaglandin E₁ synthesis, 49; for prostate, 117; suggested daily supplement, 33 (Table 5); for thyroid function, 62; for vaginal dryness, 89, 108; and vitamin A, 73, 78

About the Author

Marilyn McCusker Shannon holds a master's degree in human physiology with a minor in biochemistry from Indiana University's Medical Sciences Program. Her master's thesis involved the effects of the hormone prolactin on kidney function, a topic related to premenstrual syndrome.

She and her husband Ronald have been a teaching couple for the Couple to Couple League for Natural Family Planning since 1982. For the past six years she has also taught an undergraduate course in human anatomy and physiology at Indiana University-Purdue University at Fort Wayne, Indiana. Her interests in nutrition and reproductive health are an outgrowth of her educational background and experience as an NFP instructor.

Marilyn and Ron, a data processing professional, are the parents of a daughter, nine, and three sons, ages eleven, four and two. They are expecting their fifth child in late July, 1990. She has homeschooled the older children since their oldest started first grade. The Shannons live on a small farm outside Fort Wayne, Indiana, with a large garden and assorted sheep, chickens, cats and dogs. Their homestead is also the birthplace of their three youngest children.